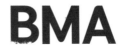

LIVING WITH FRAILTY

Increasingly, we question 'what makes us healthy?', as well as 'what makes us ill?'. What does this shift mean for frailty? Almost wholly defined in negative terms, the term 'frail' tends to refer to a group of older people who are at highest risk of adverse outcomes such as falls, infections, disability, admission to hospital or the need for long-term care. This ground-breaking book takes a holistic approach to frailty. It connects the medical literature with the wider social science discourse on ageing, and focuses on promoting wellbeing and the building up of strengths.

Living with Frailty draws together the latest biomedical evidence and good practice in this emerging area and explores ideas about assets and resilience, the role of society and the social model of disability in relation to frailty, arguing that insufficient attention is paid to positive action such as developing bone strength, maintaining good nutrition and exercising. Chapters look at:

- existing models of frailty
- person-centred care
- assessing frailty and quality of life
- how falls, and fear of falls, relate to discussions of frailty
- delirium and frailty
- the environment and frailty
- sarcopenia.

Living with Frailty is an important introduction and reference for all practitioners, researchers and students with an interest in frailty, wellbeing and social approaches to health

Shibley Rahman is a freelance researcher and aca long-term conditions, particularly frailty and dem implications of diagnosis and post-diagnostic care, a rights-based approaches. Dr Rahman's book, *Livi* award for best book for health and social care in the

LIVING WITH FRAILTY

From Assets and Deficits to Resilience

Shibley Rahman

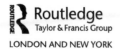

Routledge
Taylor & Francis Group

LONDON AND NEW YORK

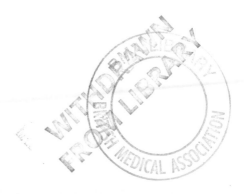

First published 2019
by Routledge
2 Park Square, Milton Park, Abingdon, Oxon OX14 4RN

and by Routledge
711 Third Avenue, New York, NY 10017

Routledge is an imprint of the Taylor & Francis Group, an informa business

British Library Cataloguing-in-Publication Data
A catalogue record for this book is available from the British Library

Library of Congress Cataloging-in-Publication Data
Names: Rahman, Shibley, author.
Title: Living with frailty: from assets and deficits to resilience / Shibley
Rahman.
Description: Abingdon, Oxon; New York, NY: Routledge, 2018. |
Includes bibliographical references and index.
Identifiers: LCCN 2018015257 | ISBN 9781138301207 (hbk) |
ISBN 9781138301214 (pbk) | ISBN 9780203732694 (ebk)
Subjects: | MESH: Frail Elderly | Chronic Disease | Frailty | Health
Promotion | Health Services for the Aged | Resilience, Psychological
Classification: LCC RB150.F37 | NLM WT 500 | DDC
616/.04780846–dc23
LC record available at https://lccn.loc.gov/2018015257

ISBN: 978-1-138-30120-7 (hbk)
ISBN: 978-1-138-30121-4 (pbk)
ISBN: 978-0-203-73269-4 (ebk)

Typeset in Bembo
by Wearset Ltd, Boldon, Tyne and Wear

Printed and bound by CPI Group (UK) Ltd, Croydon, CR0 4YY

This book is dedicated to the talented eye surgeon who restored my eyesight during the preparation of this manuscript

CONTENTS

FIGURES

TABLES

FOREWORD I

Ken Rockwood

In *Living with Frailty: from assets and deficits to resilience*, Dr. Shibley Rahman brings together much of what is known, conceptually and pragmatically, about frailty in its clinical guise. A scholar who is independent of any of the established frailty camps, Dr. Rahman aims to bring some coherence to the competing narratives about what happens to people as they age. His reading is detailed, multifaceted and perceptive, and the book can be recommended for the breadth of its consideration, and for how it challenges theoreticians and practitioners.

The central theme of his book begins to take shape as he first shows us how to take a broad view of frailty. He urges the scientific community and healthcare practitioners to be alert to its social determinants, especially those that have consequence at much younger ages across the life course than what we see in old age. Dr. Rahman also argues that we must be alert to the negative implications of the word *frailty* itself. This, he argues, is not just a matter of the pragmatics of intervention, but because we must consider ways in which frailty can be resisted by individuals. In all of this, he develops the argument that we must consider resilience as an essential goal in understanding frailty.

For someone whose research (and musings) have been so much cited in this book it might seem churlish to not simply say a few polite words of praise and move on. Instead, I see it as the greater honour to Dr. Rahman's spirit of inquiry to engage with his main argument, about resilience. Further, I know that he has read enough of my papers to recognize that I don't always agree with myself, much less anyone else. Some of this reflects an inevitable evolution in thinking. One such is the move from seeing frailty as a rules-based syndrome (of multimorbidity and disability). For me, this reached its apogee in a 1999 *Lancet* paper, which came out just as I was aiming to understand frailty more explicitly in relation to ageing [1]. That is how the notion of frailty as the accumulation of deficits arose, published in 2001 in what seemed an especially promising instance of the then up-and-coming concept of an electronic journal [2]. Working with my great friend and colleague, Arnold Mitnitski, I was taken with the many opportunities that this approach offered. One of these was a way to move from a more metaphorical understanding of the complexity of frailty to something that was susceptible to formal quantitative reasoning, while still translatable into everyday clinical care. For many years since, Arnold and I have followed the discipline that for an idea to be reasonably true, we must be able to explain it to each other, in terms that the other of us would find acceptable.

Initially we were agnostic about how deficits arose, and as Dr. Rahman notes, for a few years we put on hold the project to relate how deficits might be countered by assets, which informed my initial, words-and-diagrams model [3]. With our young geriatrician colleague Melissa Andrew, then doing her PhD, it took another six years to develop a quantitative approach that addressed the social environment – and even then, to the persisting dismay of some commentators, we again counted deficits, this time in a social vulnerability index [4].

All the while we had tried to claw our way to what we imagined was a better way to understand the origin of deficit accumulation. After some false starts, we initially settled on a deficit arising when damage could not be removed or repaired. This allowed us to invoke the apparatus of queuing theory. As anyone who has been to an airport at rush hour will know, the length of a queue is a function of the number of people arriving at the queue and how long it takes to process each one. The analogy is that the numeric value of the frailty index/length of the queue was a function of the amount of damage to which a person was exposed and their ability to repair it [5]. Each of the latter were strongly related to the degree of social vulnerability: damage is more likely in a hostile environment, and repair is more difficult [6]. To cut a long story short, subsequent work found, somewhat to our surprise, that it was possible to approximate how deficits were related to mortality without either a time-dependent damage rate or a term that specified repair: instead, these factors were simply baked into deficit accumulation [7]. The point now is not to detail every machination of this tortured and still incomplete process. Rather it is to show that those notions which seem like good ideas – I would include 'protective factors' in this [8, 9] – do not always yield to understandable quantitative reasoning.

It seems to me that sticking with a quantitative approach in understanding frailty and ageing is essential. That is because important aspects of the study of ageing oblige us to recognize that 'the problems of old age come as a package' [10, 11]. This underlies the emerging geroscience: to understand age-related disease, we must better understand what happens with ageing. One current example of how we largely fail to do that is in the failings of classic midlife epidemiology when applied to determinants of the diseases of old age. In a nutshell, the tried and true strategy of dimensionality reduction in epidemiological models is misleading in late-life epidemiology. That approach proceeds by first selecting out items (exposures/confounders/effect modifiers) that individually are statistically significant and then tests them all in a multivariable model, which reduces that candidate list further to the ones which remain when others are "controlled for". Mediation/moderation analyses are an advance, but they still do not get at this key point: small effects (even individually "insignificant" ones) still add up.

In consequence, classic midlife epidemiology gives unstable estimates. This is seen when today's risk factor is protective tomorrow. In contrast, the frailty index achieves dimensionality reduction at the level of the variable. This gives the models fewer terms and greater power.

In short, with the frailty index we quantify the size of the package of problems that accompany the diseases of old age. This we and others have demonstrated for several common diseases of old age, including dementia [12, 13] osteoporosis [14, 15], risk from the so-called 'metabolic syndrome' [16,17] and from hyponatremia [18] amongst others. Several of these papers hold across the life course, even though the relationship between the exposures and outcomes is modified by age, being strongest in younger people. A similar story emerges in heart disease [19].

For its ability to synthesize so much, and to ask penetrating questions, I recommend careful reading of Dr. Rahman's book. As with his predecessor volume on dementia [20], it will reward and stimulate.

Kenneth Rockwood, MD, FRCPC, FRCP
Professor of Medicine (Geriatric Medicine and Neurology)
Kathryn Allen Weldon Professor of Alzheimer Research
Dalhousie University
Halifax, NS, Canada

References

1 Rockwood K, Stadnyk K, MacKnight C, McDowell I, Hébert R, Hogan DB. (1999). A brief clinical instrument to classify frailty in elderly people. *Lancet*. 353(9148): 205–6.

2 Mitnitski AB, Mogilner AJ, Rockwood K. (2001). Accumulation of deficits as a proxy measure of aging. *Scientific World Journal*. August 8; 1: 323–36.

3 Rockwood K, Fox RA, Stolee P, Robertson D, Beattie BL. (1994). Frailty in elderly people: an evolving concept. *CMAJ*. 150(4): 489–95.

4 Andrew MK, Mitnitski AB, Rockwood K. (2008). Social vulnerability, frailty and mortality in elderly people. *PLoS One*. May 21; 3(5): e2232. doi:10.1371/journal.pone.0002232.

5 Mitnitski A, Song X, Rockwood K. (2013). Assessing biological aging: the origin of deficit accumulation. *Biogerontology*. December; 14(6): 709–17. doi:10.1007/s10522-013-9446-3.

6 Mitnitski A, Bao L, Rockwood K. (2006). Going from bad to worse: a stochastic model of transitions in deficit accumulation, in relation to mortality. *Mech Ageing Dev*. 127(5): 490–3.

7 Farrell SG, Mitnitski AB, Rockwood K, Rutenberg AD. (2016). Network model of human aging: frailty limits and information measures. *Phys Rev E*. November; 94(5–1): 052409.

8 Wang C, Song X, Mitnitski A, Fang X, Tang Z, Yu P, Rockwood K. (2014). Effect of health protective factors on health deficit accumulation and mortality risk in older adults in the Beijing Longitudinal Study of Aging. *J Am Geriatr Soc*. 62(5): 821–8. doi:10.1111/jgs.12792.

9 Lucicesare A, Hubbard RE, Searle SD, Rockwood K. (2010). An index of self-rated health deficits in relation to frailty and adverse outcomes in older adults. *Aging Clin Exp Res*. June; 22(3): 255–60. doi:10.3275/6625.

10 Fontana L, Kennedy BK, Longo VD, Seals D, Melov S. (2014). Medical research: treat ageing. *Nature*. July 24; 511(7510): 405–7. doi:10.1038/511405a.

11 Howlett SE, Rockwood K. (2014). Ageing: develop models of frailty. *Nature*. August 21; 512(7514): 253. doi:10.1038/512253d.

12 Song X, Mitnitski A, Rockwood K. (2011). Nontraditional risk factors combine to predict Alzheimer disease and dementia. *Neurology*. July 19; 77(3): 227–34.

13 Armstrong JJ, Mitnitski A, Andrew MK, Launer LJ, White LR, Rockwood K. (2015). Cumulative impact of health deficits, social vulnerabilities, and protective factors on cognitive dynamics in late life: a multistate modeling approach. *Alzheimers Res Ther*. June 5; 7(1): 38. doi:10.1186/s13195-015-0120-7.

14 Kennedy CC, Ioannidis G, Rockwood K, Thabane L, Adachi JD, Kirkland S, Pickard LE, Papaioannou A. (2014). A Frailty Index predicts 10-year fracture risk in adults age 25 years and older: results from the Canadian Multicentre Osteoporosis Study (CaMos). *Osteoporos Int*. December; 25(12): 2825–32. doi:10.1007/s00198-014-2828-9.

15 Li G, Ioannidis G, Pickard L, Kennedy C, Papaioannou A, Thabane L, Adachi JD. (2014). Frailty index of deficit accumulation and falls: data from the Global Longitudinal Study of Osteoporosis in Women (GLOW) Hamilton cohort. *BMC Musculoskelet Disord*. May 29; 15: 185. doi:10.1186/1471-2474-15-185.

16 Hao Q, Song X, Yang M, Dong B, Rockwood K. (2016). Understanding risk in the oldest old: frailty and the metabolic syndrome in a Chinese community sample aged 90+ years. *J Nutr Health Aging*. January; 20(1): 82–8. doi:10.1007/s12603-015-0553-5.

17 Kane AE, Gregson E, Theou O, Rockwood K, Howlett SE. (2017). The association between frailty, the metabolic syndrome, and mortality over the lifespan. *Geroscience*. 39(2): 221–9. doi:10.1007/s11357-017-9967-9.

18 Miller AJ, Theou O, McMillan M, Howlett SE, Tennankore KK, Rockwood K. (2017). Dysnatremia in relation to frailty and age in community-dwelling adults in the National Health and Nutrition Examination Survey. *J Gerontol A Biol Sci Med Sci*. March 1; 72(3): 376–81. doi:10.1093/gerona/glw114.

19 Wallace LM, Theou O, Kirkland SA, Rockwood MR, Davidson KW, Shimbo D, Rockwood K. (2014). Accumulation of non-traditional risk factors for coronary heart disease is associated with incident coronary heart disease hospitalization and death. *PLoS One*. March 13; 9(3): e90475. doi:10.1371/journal.pone.0090475.

20 Rahman S. (2017). *Enhancing health and wellbeing in dementia: a person-centred integrated care approach*. London: Jessica Kingsley Publishers.

FOREWORD II

Adam Gordon

Frailty is big news. On any given week, even a casual perusal of the health pages of any creditable media outlet will reveal multiple references to frailty. Usually such outlets use frailty as an explanator, a way of understanding why the pressures on health and social care systems are changing and evolving over time. Such analyses are frequently superficial and along the following lines: improvements in public health and individual healthcare mean people are living longer; older people are prone to frailty; people living with frailty are prone require more complicated healthcare more often; this results on unprecedented pressures on the system.

All of the above is, of course, true. The rising prevalence of frailty does have some explanatory power when it comes to understanding the challenges faced by healthcare services globally. But, as always when one scratches away beneath lay media presentations, the years of research and development in the field of frailty present us with a narrative which is much more complicated.

Frailty presents challenges and opportunities to healthcare practitioners. People with more diagnoses are more frequently frail. Frailty attenuates how medical conditions present and how they respond to treatment. Healthcare providers have, in this context, to handle multiple diagnoses in tandem and manage greater degrees of uncertainty about how each diagnosis has influenced, or is influencing, a patient's health and wellbeing. Traditional medical training focuses on gathering information from a patient, establishing a list of possible diagnoses, conducting tests to narrow the range of possible diagnoses and then starting treatment. In patients with frailty, information is harder to come by, there is frequently more than one diagnosis, and tests are often less conclusive. This means that management must proceed in the face of considerable clinical uncertainty. To do this requires specific skills and training.

Frailty presents challenges and opportunities to healthcare systems. There are questions about how best to identify frailty and at what stage in the healthcare journey to look for it. If a general practitioner has, for example, identified a patient as 'pre-frail', when and in what context should that assessment be revisited? There are questions about how best to organise systems to respond to frailty once identified. Should 'pre-habilitation' have a role in preparing older people with frailty for elective surgery? What role should case managers play and at what stage in the frailty trajectory should they become involved in care? If some aspects of frailty are reversible, how much emphasis should be placed upon systems of care to focus on slowing or reversing progression?

Frailty presents challenges and opportunities for recipients of healthcare – the public at large. There is undoubtedly stigma associated with the frailty label. Yet in clinical practice, I frequently find the conceptual model of frailty to be one that is both understood and accepted by the patients I see and their families. Both groups immediately recognise the face validity of progressive functional decline, vulnerability to minor insults, uncertainty around diagnosis and prognosis, and the need to adopt considered approaches to diagnosis and management in the face of these. Such discussions are, in my practice, often a crucial part of the groundwork for shared decision making. Yet frailty comes with negative connotations, it less than adequately describes the more positive aspects of health and wellbeing that are central to quality of life for many of my older patients and, in failing to recognise positive aspects of the ageing experience frailty could, in the wrong hands, underpin the sort of negative narratives that form the basis of ageism.

The opportunities to be realised in frailty as a concept require an understanding that goes beyond a bulletpoint in a media story about why the Emergency Department was busy. It's a complex narrative. In closing this book, Shibley Rahman talks about the Jainist proverb of the blind men and the elephant as a way of understanding frailty. The point is that it's easiest to be critical of frailty when looking at only one part of the picture. Its value is better recognised when the various ways it subtends lay and professional narratives about ageing and wellbeing are presented together. In writing this volume, Shibley hasn't shied away from complexity. He has presented both the strengths and the weaknesses of the frailty narrative. But he has presented them in a way that they can be understood, considered and evaluated. I'm not sure that, after years of providing and researching care for older people, that I can fully describe the 'frailty elephant'. I wouldn't expect that most readers will have pieced together a complete picture either by the end of this book. But the more people that understand the various parts that make up the beast, the closer we come to realising the opportunities that the years of research and development in this field present.

Adam Gordon
Clinical Associate Professor in Medicine of Older People,
University of Nottingham, UK
January 2018

PREFACE

Introduction

In a tweet,[1] Ken Rockwood (2017) reports: 'Younger people newly disabled by illness/injury often emphasized what they couldn't do. By contrast, an exemplary 80 year old amputee told me "they took my leg but I'm still here". Made an impression.' As it happens, Twitter is increasingly being used to communicate about frailty, and it has become recognised that thought leaders contribute to the conversation by promoting and disseminating frailty-related knowledge and research (Jha *et al.*, 2018).

Frailty may also be a question of outlook and expectation management. We, therefore, all need to talk about frailty. But not only that. We need to talk with the public and publicly about frailty. Living with frailty affects, and is affected by, many different aspects of a person's life (including the person's physical health, mental health, cognitive function and their social and home environment). Major drivers and incentives are being put in place to bring frailty management centre-stage in the planning cycles for the NHS and social care.

The word 'frailty' is currently defined in the Oxford English dictionary as 'the condition of being weak and delicate'.[2] A comment is then made that the word, in part, derives from the Middle English (in the sense 'weakness in morals'): from Old French *fraileté*, from Latin *fragilitas*, from *fragilis*. For those who are tech-savvie, 'Frailty Focus'[3] is a good website for general awareness about frailty for people who are frail, but there are currently limited sources of advice, support and information which can be obtained for people with frailty and families, say, compared to the national dementia charities.

I feel, personally, that much of how a person with frailty or care partners might respond to the label of frailty depends on any stigma which surrounds it. The modern idea of stigma owes a great deal to the seminal work of Erwin Goffman.

According to Erwin Goffman (1963, p. 3), stigma is an attribute that extensively discredits an individual, reducing him or her 'from a whole and usual person to a tainted, discounted one'. Stigmatising 'stereotypes' can become a basis for excluding or avoiding members of the stereotyped category. This sense of otherness is a barrier to societal inclusion. Whilst the intentions of promoting frailty are indeed well meant, the discourse brings with it significant responsibilities as well as rights.

It's great, surely, that frailty as a 'brand' is getting so much publicity, but is it all the right kind of publicity? For example, one headline ran, 'Our treatment of the frail elderly is a national scandal' (Sunday Express, 8 March 2011, cited in Manthorpe and Iliffe, 2015). There needs to be a radical shift in how frailty is presented as a health and social care issue. Last year, a senior NHS clinician, when writing on the importance of diagnosing frailty, referred to a 'crisis'. Stanley Cohen (1973) stated that moral panic happens when 'a condition, episode, person or group of persons emerges to become defined as a threat to societal values and interests'.

In international policy, the **'sustainable development goals'** agreed in March 2016 by the United Nations General Assembly set the global development agenda for the next 15 years. They include an ambitious target to reduce premature mortality from non-communicable diseases by a third by 2030. Premature mortality, defined by the World Health Organization (WHO) as deaths occurring between the ages of 15 and 70, has gained broad acceptance in health research and policy over the past decade. Such an approach, however, has been argued as being 'explicitly ageist, reflecting institutional ageism in global health policy. Its inclusion in the sustainable development goals sends a strong signal in favour of discriminating against older people in the allocation of health resources and the collection of data' (Lloyd-Sherlock et al., 2016).

It is maybe worth considering why clinicians interested in frailty are not simply 'frailogists', unless you consider that the specialty of 'frailogy' fully takes on board the striking complexity of frailty – where the rules of how conditions and their treatments in an older individual are not always easy to predict. Take, for example, how it has been argued that the respective roles of GPs and hospital specialists have become blurred, especially since the 1990s, and this is perhaps related to how GPs are taking on much of the traditional hospital care in the diagnosis and management of major diseases and even minor procedures (McManus and Hobbs, 2016). The mechanistic relationships between ageing, frailty and mortality is an important one, and worth exploring. Rutenberg and colleagues (2017) have developed a computational model in which possible health attributes are represented by the nodes of a complex network, with the connections showing a scale-free distribution. Each node can be either damaged (i.e. a deficit) or undamaged. This model arguably permits a better understanding of factors that influence the health trajectories of individuals.

It is not controversial that, in addition to biological influences, health has social determinants. For example, greater social engagement is associated with reduced disability and lower mortality (Wallace et al., 2015). Being able to identify socially frail older adults is essential for designing interventions and policy and for the prediction of health outcomes, both on the level of individual older adults and of the population (Bunt *et al.*, 2017). This book will therefore devote some time to discussing 'assets' a person who is frail might possess within himself or his community to make him more resilient, or have more 'intrinsic capacity'.

Patients with multimorbidity have complex health needs but, due to the current traditional disease-oriented approach, they face a highly fragmented form of care that leads to inefficient, ineffective and possibly harmful clinical interventions (Palmer *et al.*, 2018). This problem requires urgent attention. WHO defines Healthy Ageing 'as the process of developing and maintaining the functional ability that enables wellbeing in older age'.[4] Rather than focusing on the absence of disease, the approach considers healthy ageing from the perspective of the functional ability that enables older people to be, and to do, what they have reason to value. This ability is not only determined by an individual older person's capacities, but also by the physical and social environments they inhabit (Beard *et al.*, 2017).

A '**functional ability**' is about having the capabilities that enable all people to be and do what they have reason to value. This includes a person's ability to meet their basic needs; to learn, grow and make decisions; to be mobile; to build and maintain relationships; and to contribute to society. Functional ability is made up of the intrinsic capacity of the individual, relevant environmental characteristics and the interaction between them.

Intrinsic capacity comprises all the mental and physical capacities that a person can draw on. The level of intrinsic capacity is influenced by a number of factors such as the presence of diseases, injuries and age-related changes.

We do know that formidable barriers exist to identifying frailty, for example both in primary care, in hospital and other settings (see Figure P.1).

But some attention will inevitably have to be given as to the ultimate clinical trajectories. I will return to this issue in Chapter 7 when I discuss person-centred integrated care. In response to a clinician sharing information with a patient that he or she is 'severely frail', that patient might legitimately want to know what might be coming next? Not everyone might be found to be 'progressively dwindling' (a well known and respected term), and yet such framing of the narrative might expose a person who is frail to yet further institutional vulnerability.

David Oliver moots: 'Once you're progressively dwindling you're likely to become more dependent, be admitted and readmitted more frequently, lose function or weight in hospital, and die, even when care is sensitive and skilled' (Oliver, 2017).

With a highly developed healthcare system supporting us to later life, it is reasonable that clinicians can be expected to cope when frailty declares itself as a health or social care crisis. However, we must also recognise that this is a long-term condition, which can predate crisis by a decade or more (Vernon, 2016). Whilst as such a crisis is not an issue for 'blame', there is clearly a debate to be had whether community assets have been mobilised adequately for a frail older person living on her own with a sedentary lifestyle and poor nutrition. There is a need to integrate predominantly medically driven understandings of frailty within a wider conceptual

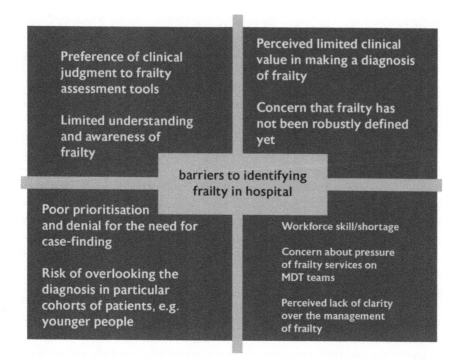

FIGURE P.1 Thematic analysis of survey free-text comments regarding barriers to identifying frailty in hospital

Source: based on Figure 1, page 210 of Taylor JK, Fox J, Shah P, Ali A, Hanley M, Hyatt R.
(2017). Barriers to the identification of frailty in hospital: a survey of UK clinicians. *Future Hosp J.*
October 1; 4(3): 207–12. doi:10.7861/futurehosp.4-3-207.

framework (Nicholson *et al.*, 2017). Research on the factors associated with or
predicting a spontaneous reversion from frailty are still inconclusive. Results from
available studies on possible sex differences are conflicting.

Currently, Health Education England is responsible for delivering a better health
and healthcare workforce nationally and locally, and is responsible for the education, training and personal development of staff, including recruiting for values.
Whilst there have been significant improvements over the last few years in the
acute care response to older people, there is much to understand how exactly the
needs of people who are frail, and their care partners, can be addressed in the 'right
place, right way, and right time'. Arguably it is the technology to which geriatricians can usefully contribute to or even coordinate – Comprehensive Geriatric
Assessment (CGA).[5]

Dissemination, as well as the discovery, of optimal practice is therefore to be
encouraged. The Acute Frailty Network seeks to bring together centres from across
the country to share best practice in developing urgent care solutions for frail older
people. The focus is on the first 72 hours in acute hospitals, whilst maintaining

strong relationships with, and awareness of, the broader system (Conroy, 2015). The Acute Frailty Network brings together an effective blend of practical expertise and experience to support organisations to successfully implement and improve Acute Frailty Services locally.[6] The challenge in the immediate future is implementing in a cogent way a meaningful response to the notion of 'intrinsic capacity'. As introduced above, intrinsic capacity has been defined as the composite of all the physical and mental capacities that an individual can draw on (Beard et al., 2016).

Frailty is becoming more common due to an ageing population. Frailty might be perceived as the age-related decline of physiological systems determining the reduction of intrinsic capacity, consequently leading to increased risk of negative health outcomes (Cesari, 2017). Multimorbidity is a common and important phenomenon which may affect quality of life, increase medical needs and make people live more years of life with disability. Negative outcomes related to multimorbidity occur beyond what we would expect from the summed effect of single conditions, as chronic diseases interact with each other (Vetrano et al., 2017).

About this book

This book comprises a number of chapters (listed in Box P.1) on specific important contemporary topics (not including this one or the Afterword). It is intended to reflect the current literature, as peer-reviewed and published globally to date (early 2018), there were inevitably space constraints; for example, I should like to have included a chapter on other topics including managing medication in frailty.

BOX P.1

Preface
Chapter 1 Frailty: from awareness to identity
Chapter 2 Living well with frailty: from identity to care
Chapter 3 Evidence-based practice in frailty: falls and activity
Chapter 4 Surgical outcomes, cognitive frailty and delirium
Chapter 5 Sarcopenia and frailty
Chapter 6 Interventions in frailty care and enhancing independence
Chapter 7 Person-centred integrated care and end of life
Afterword

Although frailty becomes more common as people get older, it is not an inevitable consequence of ageing and can be applicable in all age groups. To balance the narrative regarding frailty, it's perhaps imperative that assets should be given due weight. Assets can be described as the collective resources which individuals and communities have at their disposal, which protect against negative health outcomes and promote health status. An asset-based approach makes visible and values the skills, knowledge, connections and potential in a community. It promotes capacity, connectedness and social capital. Asset based approaches emphasise the need to redress the balance between meeting needs and nurturing the strengths and resources of people and communities. A person's frailty can change (up or down) over time. It is vital to know how to enrol the person with frailty in post-assessment care and support planning and associated interventions. Shropshire CCG[7] has supported a programme to recruit and train practice-based volunteers who help connect patients with voluntary and community sector services. Social prescribing might help, and involves the referral of patients with needs to local services and activities provided by the third sector (community, voluntary and social enterprise sector); it aims to promote partnership working between the health and the social sector to address the wider determinants of health (Pescheny, Pappas and Randhawa, 2018).

Dawn Moody, in a blogpost on the NHS England website,[8] introduces the notion of a 'frailty fulcrum'. The **'frailty fulcrum'** highlights the multidimensional nature of frailty. It considers the many different aspects of our lives that contribute to our overall wellbeing through a series of domains. The domains identified in the model are:

- Social environment, including communities;
- Physical environment;
- Psychological status, which includes both specific conditions, such as anxiety, or more general feelings like confidence, fear or motivation;
- Long-term conditions, e.g. organ failure, cognitive impairment;
- Acute health problems, including for example, infection;
- Systems of care.

I feel this 'frailty fulcrum' nicely parallels the narrative of my book, exploring assets, deficits and resilience. One 'asset', for example, might be to boost confidence to overcome through cognitive behavioural therapy the 'fear of falling' which leads to a decline in daily physical activity, quality of life, a change in gait parameters and an increased risk of falling; see Chapter 3. Instead of thinking about people in terms of the value they bring to society, the narrative becomes one of their economic 'cost' to society. It's only a short leap to outright ageism. As elegantly argued by Romero-Ortuno and O'Shea (2013), it can be difficult to place people on the 'frailty continuum'. Whilst wellbeing is not simply the absence of ill-being, according to the current quality of life research anyway, it is reasonable to view people as lying on a continuum between 'fitness' and 'frailty'.

In frailty, it is usually the number of things that have 'gone wrong' that is more important than the exact nature of the individual problems (examples of 'problems' may include poor vision, hearing or mobility, loneliness, history of falls and memory loss, as well as diagnosed long-term physical and mental health conditions). But the wider environment is absolutely critical. Environments include the home, community and broader society, and all the factors within them such as the built environment, people and their relationships, attitudes and values, health and social policies, the systems that support them and the services that they implement. The causal role of social conditions in the great variations in the quality of life of older individuals within a country – as well as across countries – raises profound questions of social justice and social action (Venkatapuram *et al.*, 2017). There is a compelling argument now for mainstreaming assets into policy such as dementia friendly communities, for example (Rahman and Swaffer, 2018).

A profoundly significant contribution has been to argue that frailty can be considered in relation to 'deficit accumulation', ultimately from Ken Rockwood and his colleagues. Recalling that frailty is an age-associated, nonspecific vulnerability, this powerful contribution considers the symptoms, signs, diseases and disabilities as deficits, which are combined in a frailty index (Rockwood and Mitnitski, 2007). Targeting potentially modifiable aspects of frailty preoperatively, such as improving functional status, may improve peri-operative outcomes and decrease readmissions (Wahl *et al.*, 2017). It seems that the rate of increase in the accumulation of deficits is an estimate of the rate of ageing, and, in general, the 'frailty index' characterises individual health across the fitness-frailty continuum from the fittest to the frailest (Mitnitski *et al.*, 2013). The beauty about focusing on deficits is that the narrative does have a genuine biological underpinning. For example, molecular identification of genomic instability may help to anticipate recognition of individuals who are frail (Sánchez-Flores *et al.*, 2018). Biomarkers, once identified reliably, might be of clinical utility in spotting people who are 'pre-frail'. Given its sensitivity, specificity, objectivity and predictive capacity, several authors have pointed out that cellular and molecular biomarkers may potentially be used for frailty identification; however, to date, no specific biological marker has been identified as a definitive marker for frailty.

Running an 'over-intellectualised' approach may, however, miss a bigger picture, and, by pursuing an over-medicalised approach to frailty, we are in real danger of ignoring other aspects of a person's wellbeing. There is evidence that older people may not recognise themselves as being frail, or want to be considered as such, even if they are happy to accept that they are an older person; see for example the BGS' 'Fit for frailty' report for a brief discussion (British Geriatrics Society/RCGP/Age UK, 2014).[9] Respondents to a recent survey by Age UK universally regarded 'frail' as a negative label. People with stigmatised conditions like this can be so ashamed of talking about them that they are unable to seek help. The repercussions are serious. Failure to seek care can worsen symptoms. Frailty is an age-related syndrome described as the decreased ability of an organism to respond to stressors (shown in Figure P.2). A number of epidemiological studies have reported that frailty increases the risk of future cognitive decline and that cognitive impairment increases the risk of frailty, suggesting that cognition and frailty interact within a cycle of decline associated with ageing (Robertson *et al.*, 2013).

Multiprofessional and multi-agency working will increasingly need to support work that ensures that people can benefit from more person-centred but also more efficient, safer care.[10] The development of new roles for nurses, radiographers and pharmacists have supported a more efficient approach to meeting the needs of

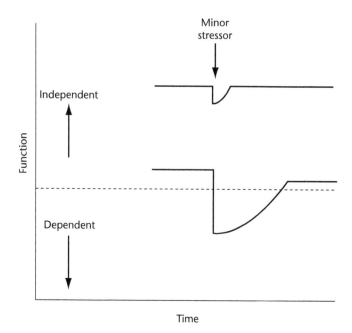

FIGURE P.2 Vulnerability of frail elderly people to a sudden change in health status after a minor illness

Source: redrawn from Figure 1, p. 753 of Clegg A, Young J, Iliffe S, Rikkert MO, Rockwood K. (2013). Frailty in elderly people. *Lancet*. March 2; 381(9868): 752–62. doi:10.1016/S0140-6736(12)62167-9. Epub 2013 February 8.

Note
The upper line represents a fit elderly individual who, after a minor stressor event such as an infection, has a small deterioration in function but then recovers fully. The lower line represents a frail elderly individual who, after a similar stressor event, undergoes a larger deterioration, which may manifest as functional dependency, and who does not return to baseline homoeostasis.

people who may previously have had to be seen by a medical practitioner (NHS Scotland, 2016).

The discussion about frailty could and should, therefore, be framed, arguably, as well in terms of boosting assets – eating healthily to build up resilience, for example, or exercise training before surgery to prevent postoperative confusion, or eating a diet and boosting self-confidence so that you might be at lower risk of falls and fractures. Take for example sarcopenia, which can contribute to frailty. Sarcopenia is defined as an age associated decline in skeletal muscle mass. The pathophysiology of sarcopenia is multifactorial, with decreased caloric intake, muscle fibre denervation, intracellular oxidative stress, hormonal decline and enhanced myostatin signaling all thought to contribute (Marty *et al.*, 2017). There is a new and emerging knowledge of pharmacological interventions that can be used to enhance the well-being of people living with frailty, which we ignore at our peril. Trials with various agents, including selective androgen receptor modulators and myostatin inhibitors, show promise as future treatment options. Myostatin blockers include myostatin-blocking antibodies, myostatin propeptide, follistatin and follistatin-related proteins, soluble myostatin receptors, small interfering RNA and small chemical inhibitors (Tsuchida, 2008). I discuss sarcopenia in Chapter 6.

In general, health and social care professionals might benefit from shifting their mindset from thinking about 'people *with frailty*' to '*people with* frailty', and walking within the community rather than viewing all patients as patients, service users or consumers. Although rising numbers of people are dying in very old age, relatively little is known about symptom control for 'older old' people or whether care in different settings enables them to die comfortably (Fleming *et al.*, 2017). And, ideally, we should use language which reflects this. This means participating in conversations that resonate with people, and trying harder to remind people that living with frailty is not an inevitable or irreversible part of getting older. It is possible to maintain independence by engaging with services.

Further reading

This book is merely a snapshot of the current field of frailty. It is worth emphasising that this book is not to be used as a source of professional advice, but that this book is a contemporaneous academic review. The best way to use this book is to analyse critically the evolving field of frailty from a multidisciplinary, sophisticated perspective, and not to use it as a source of professional advice. The field of frailty is now fast moving, and you are encouraged to read around widely, including high quality journals such as Age and Ageing,[11] the *Journal of Frailty and Aging*,[12] *Geriatrics*,[13] and *BMC Medicine*.[14] You might also like blogposts by Dawn Moody at NHS England.[15]

Two other recent developments are also noteworthy. NIHR's *Comprehensive Care*,[16] looks at the evidence behind the concept of 'frailty' in older people living in hospital. Also, Health Education England (HEE) and NHS England have commissioned the development of a Frailty Core Capabilities Framework.[17] The framework will provide a single, consistent and comprehensive framework on which to base review and development of staff. The framework aims to describe core capabilities, i.e. knowledge, skills and behaviours which are common and transferable across different types of service provision – including health, social care, local government and housing sectors.

Good luck and enjoy the journey!

Dr Shibley Rahman
Queen's Scholar
BA(Hons), MA, MB, BChir, PhD (all Cambridge)
MRCP (UK)
LLB (BPP Law School), LLM (University of Law of England and Wales)
MBA (BPP Business School)
PgDipLaw (BPP Law School)
London
January 2018

Notes

1 https://twitter.com/Krockdoc/status/947084164968402944.
2 https://en.oxforddictionaries.com/definition/frailty.
3 www.frailtyfocus.nhs.uk.
4 www.who.int/ageing/healthy-ageing/en.
5 www.bgs.org.uk/april-new-15/newsletter/news-april15/apr15-afn-conroy.
6 www.acutefrailtynetwork.org.uk.
7 www.england.nhs.uk/wp-content/uploads/2016/03/releas-capcty-case-study-8-70.pdf.
8 www.england.nhs.uk/blog/dawn-moody.
9 www.bgs.org.uk/campaigns/fff/fff2_full.pdf.
10 www.england.nhs.uk/wp-content/uploads/2015/01/mdt-dev-guid-flat-fin.pdf.
11 https://academic.oup.com/ageing.
12 www.jfrailtyaging.com.
13 www.mdpi.com/journal/geriatrics/editors.
14 www.springer.com/medicine/journal/12916?detailsPage=editorialBoard.
15 www.england.nhs.uk/author/dr-dawn-moody.
16 www.dc.nihr.ac.uk/themed-reviews/comprehensive-care.htm.
17 www.skillsforhealth.org.uk/services/item/607-frailty-core-capabilities-framework.

References

Beard JR, Araujo de Carvalho I, Sumi Y, Officer A, Thiyagarajan JA. (2017). Healthy ageing: moving forward. *Bull World Health Organ.* November 1; 95(11): 730–730A. doi:10.2471/BLT.17.203745.

Beard JR, Officer A, de Carvalho IA, Sadana R, Pot AM, Michel JP, Lloyd-Sherlock P, Epping Jordan JE, Peeters GMEEG, Mahanani WR, Thiyagarajan JA, Chatterji S. (2016). The World report on ageing and health: a policy framework for healthy ageing. *Lancet.* May 21; 387(10033): 2145–54. doi:10.1016/S0140-6736(15)00516-4. Epub 2015 October 29.

British Geriatrics Society/RCGP/Age UK. (2014). Fit for frailty: Part 1. Consensus best practice guidance for the care of older people living in community and outpatient settings. www.bgs.org.uk/campaigns/fff/fff_full.pdf.

Bunt S, Steverink N, Andrew MK, Schans CPV, Hobbelen H. (2017). Cross-cultural adaptation of the Social Vulnerability Index for use in the Dutch context. *Int J Environ Res Public Health.* November 14; 14(11). pii: E1387. doi:10.3390/ijerph14111387.

Cesari M. (2017). Intersections between frailty and the concept of intrinsic capacity. *Innovation in Aging.* July 1; 1(1): 692. https://doi.org/10.1093/geroni/igx004.2479.

Cohen S. (1973). *Folk devils and moral panics: the creation of the mods and rockers.* London: Paladin.

Conroy S. (2015). The Acute Frailty Network: solutions for urgent care for older people? March 16. https://britishgeriatricssociety.wordpress.com/2015/03/19/the-acute-frailty-network-solutions-for-urgent-care-for-older-people.

Fleming J, Calloway R, Perrels A, Farquhar M, Barclay S, Brayne C; Cambridge City over-75s Cohort (CC75C) study. (2017). Dying comfortably in very old age with or without dementia in different care settings: a representative 'older old' population study. *BMC Geriatr.* October 5; 17(1): 222. doi:10.1186/s12877-017-0605-2.

Goffman E. (1963). *Stigma: notes on the management of spoiled identity.* Englewood Cliffs, N.J: Prentice-Hall.

Jha SR, McDonagh J, Prichard R, Newton PJ, Hickman LD, Fung E, Macdonald PS, Ferguson C. (2018). #Frailty: a snapshot Twitter report on frailty knowledge translation. *Australas J Ageing.* May 7. doi:10.1111/ajag.12540. [Epub ahead of print].

Lloyd-Sherlock PG, Ebrahim S, McKee M, Prince MJ. (2016). Institutional ageism in global health policy. *BMJ*. August 31; 354: i4514. doi:10.1136/bmj.i4514.

Manthorpe J, Iliffe S. (2015). Frailty – from bedside to buzzword? *Journal of Integrated Care*, 23(3): 120–8. https://doi.org/10.1108/JICA-01-2015-0007.

Marty E, Liu Y, Samuel A, Or O, Lane J. (2017). A review of sarcopenia: enhancing aware-ness of an increasingly prevalent disease. *Bone*. December; 105: 276–86. doi:10.1016/j.bone.2017.09.008. Epub 2017 September 18.

McManus RJ, Hobbs FD. (2016). Should general practice be a specialty in its own right? *BMJ*. September 27; 354: i5097. doi:10.1136/bmj.i5097.

Mitnitski A, Song X, Rockwood K. (2013). Assessing biological aging: the origin of deficit accumulation. *Biogerontology*. December; 14(6): 709–17. doi:10.1007/s10522-013-9446-3. Epub 2013 July 17.

NHS Scotland. (2016). *Realistic medicine*. Chief Medical Officer's Annual Report 2015–16. www.hi-netgrampian.org/wp-content/uploads/2017/03/Realistic-Medicine-Report-Feb-2017.pdf.

Nicholson C, Gordon AL, Tinker A. (2017). Changing the way 'we' view and talk about frailty. *Age Ageing*. May 1; 46(3): 349–51. doi:10.1093/ageing/afw224.

Oliver D. (2017). 'Progressive dwindling', frailty, and realistic expectations. *BMJ*. September 5; 358: j3954. doi:10.1136/bmj.j3954.

Palmer K, Marengoni A, Forjaz MJ, Jureviciene E, Laatikainen T, Mammarella F, Muth C, Navickas R, Prados-Torres A, Rijken M, Rothe U, Souchet L, Valderas J, Vontetsianos T, Zaletel J, Onder G; Joint Action on Chronic Diseases and Promoting Healthy Ageing Across the Life Cycle (JA-CHRODIS). (2018). Multimorbidity care model: recom-mendations from the consensus meeting of the Joint Action on Chronic Diseases and Promoting Healthy Ageing across the Life Cycle (JA-CHRODIS). *Health Policy*. January; 122(1): 4–11. doi:10.1016/j.healthpol.2017.09.006. Epub 2017 September 14.

Pescheny JV, Pappas Y, Randhawa G. (2018). Facilitators and barriers of implementing and delivering social prescribing services: a systematic review. *BMC Health Serv Res*. February 7; 18(1): 86. doi:10.1186/s12913-018-2893-4.

Rahman S, Swaffer K. (2018). Assets-based approaches and dementia-friendly com-munities. *Dementia* (London). January 1. doi:10.1177/1471301217751533. [Epub ahead of print].

Robertson DA, Savva GM, Kenny RA. (2013). Frailty and cognitive impairment: a review of the evidence and causal mechanisms. *Ageing Res Rev*. September; 12(4): 840–51. doi:10.1016/j.arr.2013.06.004. Epub 2013 July 4.

Rockwood K, Mitnitski A. (2007). Frailty in relation to the accumulation of deficits. *J Ger-ontol A Biol Sci Med Sci*. July; 62(7): 722–7.

Romero-Ortuno R, O'Shea D. (2013). Fitness and frailty: opposite ends of a challenging continuum! Will the end of age discrimination make frailty assessments an imperative? *Age Ageing*. May; 42(3): 279–80. doi:10.1093/ageing/afs189. Epub 2013 January 24.

Rutenberg AD, Mitnitski AB, Farrell SG, Rockwood K. (2017). Unifying aging and frailty through complex dynamical networks. *Exp Gerontol*. August 25. pii: S0531–5565(17)30482-5. doi:10.1016/j.exger.2017.08.027. [Epub ahead of print].

Sánchez-Flores M, Marcos-Pérez D, Lorenzo-López L, Maseda A, Millán-Calenti JC, Bonassi S, Pásaro E, Laffon B, Valdiglesias V. (2018). Frailty syndrome and genomic instability in older adults: suitability of the Cytome Micronucleus Assay as a diagnostic tool. *J Gerontol A Biol Sci Med Sci*. January 13. doi:10.1093/gerona/glx258. [Epub ahead of print].

Tsuchida K. (2008). Myostatin inhibition by a follistatin-derived peptide ameliorates the pathophysiology of muscular dystrophy model mice. *Acta Myol*. July; 27: 14–18.

Venkatapuram S, Ehni HJ, Saxena A. (2017). Equity and healthy ageing. *Bull World Health Organ*. November 1; 95(11): 791–2. doi:10.2471/BLT.16.187609. Epub 2017 September 18.

Vernon, M. (2016). Why is diagnosing frailty important? NHS England blog, 19 September. www.england.nhs.uk/blog/martin-vernon-2.

Vetrano DL, Calderón-Larrañaga A, Marengoni A, Onder G, Bauer JM, Cesari M, Ferrucci L, Fratiglioni L. (2017). An international perspective on chronic multimorbidity: approaching the elephant in the room. *J Gerontol A Biol Sci Med Sci*. September 16. doi:10.1093/gerona/glx178. [Epub ahead of print].

Wahl TS, Graham LA, Hawn MT, Richman J, Hollis RH, Jones CE, Copeland LA, Burns EA, Itani KM, Morris MS. (2017). Association of the Modified Frailty Index with 30-day surgical readmission. *JAMA Surg*. August 1; 152(8): 749–57. doi:10.1001/jamasurg.2017.1025.

Wallace LM, Theou O, Pena F, Rockwood K, Andrew MK. (2015). Social vulnerability as a predictor of mortality and disability: cross-country differences in the survey of health, aging, and retirement in Europe (SHARE). *Aging Clin Exp Res*. June; 27(3): 365–72. doi:10.1007/s40520-014 0271-6. Epub 2014 September 12.

ACKNOWLEDGEMENTS

Thanks to Professor Matteo Cesari (Associate Professor, Primary Università degli Studi di Milano Milan, Italy), and Dr Zoe Wyrko (Consultant physician at University Hospital, Birmingham) for reading through the manuscript prior to publication.

I am also grateful to Professors Ken Rockwood (Professor of Medicine (Geriatric Medicine and Neurology) at Dalhousie University, Nova Scotia, Canada) and Adam Gordon (Clinical Associate Professor in Medicine of Older People, Faculty of Medicine and Health Sciences, Nottingham, UK) for reading through the manuscript, and for generously writing the Forewords to this book.

Finally, I should like to thank NIHR Dissemination Centre for their excellent recent 'Comprehensive Care: Older people living with frailty in hospitals' review (www.dc.nihr.ac.uk/themed-reviews/Comprehensive-Care-final.pdf), and also Skills for Health for their work on the 'Frailty Core Capabilities Framework' (www.skillsforhealth.org.uk/services/item/607-frailty-core-capabilities-framework). Whilst this book is not intended as a textbook for the 'Frailty Core Capabilities Framework', I hope that the research and evidence presented will stimulate informed practice and discussion for all practitioners in frailty, including allied health professionals and geriatricians of all training grades.

1

FRAILTY

From awareness to identity

Aim

In this chapter, I'd like to look at what frailty actually is, and how its identity is rather ambiguous when considering whether it is a description of health or illness. I will briefly review methods for its measurement, and consider how a more holistic view of frailty necessitates a consideration of health and community assets and capabilities, as well as deficits.

Introduction

> Research can be like panning for gold: you go through a lot of dirt before you find a nugget that can be useful.

Frailty is a complex and multidimensional state linked to other concepts including multimorbidity, disability, dependency and personal resilience. Understanding what frailty *actually is* has come on leaps and bounds, and this means we are now in a position to raise awareness of it. The 'accumulated deficits approach', a highly respected model (*and rightly so*), tends to be emphasised most of all, but it is increasingly clear that a narrative simply based on deficits cannot give the complete story, perhaps. An understanding of deficits is necessary but not sufficient. Scientific progress in frailty has been arguably somewhat hampered, however, by the lack of consensus on its definition, which in turn delays development of screening and diagnostic tools, as well as treatment (Rodríguez-Mañas et al., 2013). Some progress, however, has been made in recent years. Frailty, notwithstanding, is a complex interplay of a person's assets and deficits as a result of the combination of factors such as age, gender, lifestyle, socioeconomic background, comorbidities and affective, cognitive or sensory issues (Lang et al., 2009; Rockwood and Hubbard, 2004).

All these factors have to be put into the 'melting pot' if we are to understand how frailty develops.

In thinking about one's reaction to 'frail persons', it is impossible to ignore that various examples in the 1960s represented a potent expression of a deep political and social disaffection at certain identities (Bayer, 2008). It was within this context that we must understand the powerful impact of Erving Goffman's work *Stigma* (1963) that spoke powerfully of individuals who stood as 'discredited person[s] facing an unaccepting world' (p. 19). In medicine, there is a tradition of presenting certainty about the diagnosis. The danger of presenting 'frail elders' as an underclass with no rights, to be oppressed, is a very nasty one. In domains of medicine, there is a sense of 'scientificness' to the activities of diagnosing that imbue the term of 'diagnosis' with a kind of reverence (Hayne, 2003). Acquiring a medical diagnosis is often accompanied by a sense of having been seen through 'officially' by 'one' who truly knows and in an authoritative way can pronounce on one's state of functioning. But labelling someone with a diagnosis can also have its problems and unintended consequences. For example, Bjorklund (1996) suggests that receiving a psychiatric diagnosis goes much beyond acquiring knowledge about functioning, in that the diagnostic label becomes a 'transforming influence' actually to shape 'present and future life expectations' (p. 1329).

Deficit models focus on identifying problems and needs of populations requiring professional skills and resources, potentially resulting in high levels of dependence on hospital, social care and welfare services. They can therefore be financially costly. In contrast, **asset models** tend to accentuate positive ability, strengths, capability and capacity to identify problems and activate solutions, which promote the self-esteem and motivation of individuals and communities, leading to less reliance on professional services. In reality, of course, both are important – one needs to redress the balance between the more dominant 'deficit model' and the less well known (and perhaps less well understood) 'asset model'.

Labelling services as 'frailty hubs' with 'frailty checklists' may, of course, pull the pendulum away from the person to the power of the diagnostic label and the 'disease entity'. So the narrative inadvertently becomes one of 'frailty in bed six', away from personhood. But the depersonalisation and 'efficiency' of modern medicine are often blamed on ever mounting time pressures and a focus on delivering technically appropriate evidence-based care (Chochinov *et al.*, 2015). Lay and professional literature converge upon a common theme, that people do not want to be treated merely as diseases. Various movements, such as dignity-centred medicine, spirituality and health, and palliative care, have rightly been advocating for more whole-person models of care (Puchalski and Jafari, 2015).

This, I feel, is in fact a central issue in the development of the 'frailty concept'.

Frailty has been recognised as an important condition by the Institute of Medicine and the European Union, although a consensus conference held in 2011 concluded that, while frailty has a clear conceptual framework and is useful in clinical settings, there is no single operational definition of frailty that can satisfy all experts and more research is needed (Orlando Frailty Reference Group, 2013). Seeing individuals as a whole person, with both mental and physical health needs and social needs, will arguably deliver better patient care and improved outcomes. Leading an engaging, meaningful and satisfying life is an essential part of '**successful ageing**' (Rowe and Kahn, 1998; Rowe and Kahn, 2015; Steptoe *et al.*, 2015). Up until the 1960s, the prevailing theories of the ageing process considered older age to be a progressive, linear decline towards death (Cumming, 1968). Studies into contributors of 'successful ageing' highlighted instead healthy lifestyle (physical activity, nutrition), environmental enrichment and stress avoidance, and methods to preserve cognitive function by measures that promote neuronal plasticity (Woo, Leung and Zhang, 2016). The use of the word 'successful' is fraught with difficulties, as the opposite implies failure and potentially fault, so a narrative of **healthy ageing** has emerged.

Current healthcare systems are built around the traditional paradigm of patients diagnosed with a single acute illness, and don't deal with complexity or multimorbidity well. They are, therefore arguably, largely unprepared to face the increasing demands from patients arising from the expansion of an older population with specific medical needs related to *multiple* chronic disorders (Le Lain *et al.*, 2017). Geriatricians, in contrast, largely see frailty as an individual's increased risk of adverse outcomes; this risk often varies with age (Howlett and Rockwood, 2013). 'Frailty' is a long established clinical expression that implies concern about an elderly person's vulnerability and outlook (Clegg *et al.*, 2013), but there has perhaps been a striking reluctance to scrutinise what *precisely* makes patients 'resilient'. Modern healthcare now needs to reconcile itself to complex patients (Rockwood and Hubbard, 2004). Because older adults are more likely than younger individuals to have complex care needs which affect daily living, this population has increasingly become a priority target group to receive and benefit from integrated **person-centred care** (Kogan *et al.*, 2016).

A person living with frailty is not simply the sum of constituent organ-specific failures. Despite an increase in interest in frailty, the pathophysiological changes underlying and preceding frailty are not clearly or fully understood yet. Inflammation is one such potential pathophysiological change which may be closely linked with frailty (Chen *et al.*, 2014). Pro-inflammatory cytokines may influence frailty, either directly by promoting protein degradation, or indirectly by affecting important metabolic pathways (Lang *et al.*, 2009). The association of inflammation with frailty seems consistent across different frailty definitions (Hubbard *et al.*, 2015). Thus, inflammation-related biomarkers might be powerful predictors of frailty and mortality in the elderly (DeMartinis *et al.*, 2006), and this phenomenon is referred to as '**inflamm-aging**' (Franceschi *et al.*, 2000).

The case for better awareness of people living with frailty and of their care partners

There is, as yet, no multimillion pound campaign run by a big charity called 'Frailty friends'. Heightened awareness, together with financial constraints, give an opportunity to develop cost-effective, high-quality care for 'older' people, resulting in better outcomes and an improvement in long-term care planning. Ongoing research programmes, together with developing productive networks, ties and collaborations, might possibly lead, in time, to a portfolio of tools or instruments to aid the non-specialist in recognising and managing patients who are frail (Wyrko, 2015). Not everyone of the same age has the same risk of adverse health outcomes. The greater vulnerability of some people compared with others of the same chronological age is best understood through frailty. But there has been an element of accelerating momentum to 'deal with frailty' through the generation of a *moral panic* reminiscent of other previous health issues: for example, 'by attacking AIDS-related stigma, we create a social climate conducive to a rational, effective, and compassionate response to this epidemic' (Herek and Glunt, 1988, p. 890).

The potential link between frailty and cognitive and affective processes is of interest in the context of what has been described as the '**frailty identity crisis**'. This sense of 'crisis' has been proposed to occur when challenging transitions from independence to frailty are accompanied by somewhat maladaptive psychological responses (Fillit and Butler, 2009). Affected individuals are said to experience a crisis of identity and a decline in psychological wellbeing, as they are faced with losses in health and independence that mark the transition from fitness to frailty. This is a provocative idea which has to date received relatively little empirical attention, and surprisingly so (Andrew *et al.*, 2012). The similarity to what happens on a disclosure of dementia diagnosis is striking. People at a particular age who, in consequence of multisystem impairments, are at higher risk of dying are said to be 'frail' while those at lower risk are said to be 'fit' (Clegg *et al.*, 2013). **Self-determination** can be defined as a process in which a person has both control and ethical/legal rights, and has the ability and knowledge to make decisions of his/her own free choice. The possibility to exercise self-determination in daily life is also an important condition for older people's subjective health and wellbeing and an ability to exercise independence (Ottenvall Hammar *et al.*, 2014). Geriatric syndromes are associated with poor quality of life and negative health outcomes. Their management is today challenging, so that recognising pathophysiological mechanisms and associated factors might help physicians to deal better with them (Vetrano *et al.*, 2016).

Fewer social resources (e.g. smaller social networks, loneliness and lack of social support) are associated with negative ageing perceptions (Steverink *et al.*, 2001) and frailty (Gobbens *et al.*, 2010; Woo *et al.*, 2005). In practical terms, it is fundamental to know what support, services and resources are available for families and care partners, including practical and emotional support services, and know how to access them (see, for example, 'Support for carers' from 'Frailty Focus'[1]), or how to arrange a 'carer's assessment' under the Care Act 2014.[2]

The Care Act 2014 gives local authorities a responsibility to assess a carer's need for support, where the carer appears to have such needs.[3] When the carer's assessment is complete, the local authority must decide whether the carer's needs are eligible for support from the local authority. There is, however, a potential for dilemmas arising where there are differing needs and priorities between people living with frailty and their carers; these have already been clearly articulated for dementia.[4] In the community, 'personalised health and care' might be promoted through the use of personal health budgets (see, for example, NHS England, 'Personal Health Budgets'[5]), and devices such as lasting powers of attorney for health and financial decisions might be important for carers if persons living with frailty lose mental capacity.

In reality, hospitals only see a *glimpse* of a person's state of health and illness but engulf a huge proportion of financial resources. The growing number of visits is being made by older adults, who present with a greater level of complexity and urgency more often than younger individuals and who use more resources and stay longer during a visit in the emergency department (McCusker *et al.*, 2012). Traditional emergency medicine facilities, staff training and behaviours have tended to focus upon '**clinically urgent scenarios**', creating a potential mis-match between the emergency department response and the nature of the population that they are increasingly facing (Conroy and Turpin, 2016). Originally emergency departments

> were designed and organised to treat and care for patients with a single acute illness. However, a large proportion of older patients suffer from multiple chronic diseases. In addition, the early identification of frail older patients as part of standard of care appears to be difficult in a emergency setting due to the hectic work environment.
>
> *(Brouwers* et al.*, 2017, p. 335)*

Possible key components of a 'frailty-friendly' emergency department are shown in Table 1.1.

TABLE 1.1 Components of a 'frail friendly emergency department'

Environmental adaptations	Access to visual and hearing aids (e.g. portable amplifiers), large print information Clear signage Non-skid flooring and hand rails
Screening and referral	Specialist nurse involvement with the use of screening tools for geriatric syndromes such as delirium, falls, immobility, polypharmacy
Improved transitions	Rapid access to social work Multidisciplinary team based in the emergency department Telephone follow-up system Care of the elderly follow-up clinic
Staff education	Specialist training programmes for staff working in the Emergency Department relating to geriatric patients and their differences in the emergency setting Frailty capabilities framework

Source: adapted from Conroy and Turpin, 2016, p. 582, table 1.

What is frailty?

But what exactly is 'frailty'? This is not an easy question at all, and is at the heart of this book. Frailty may be viewed as a syndrome involving some decline with ageing; dysregulation of the endocrine, metabolic and immune systems; and common age-related chronic diseases, representing a continuum from normal ageing to a final state of disability and death (Woo et al., 2012). It is thus conceptualised as the transitional state between robustness and functional decline (Lang, Michel and Zekry, 2009). In frailty, there is '**homeostenosis**'; that is, a decreased ability to maintain homeostasis in times of acute stress (Ahmed et al., 2007). Rockwood previously suggested criteria for a successful definition of frailty, including content validity (i.e. it is dynamic, includes multiple determinants and is useful in different situations), construct validity (i.e. more common in women and advancing age and related to disability) and criterion validity (i.e. predicts adverse outcomes including mortality) (Rockwood, 2005).

A **long-term condition** (LTC) is defined as: 'a condition that cannot, at present, be cured but can be controlled by medication and/or other treatment/ therapies' (Department of Health, 2012). The commonest LTCs (e.g. chronic obstructive pulmonary disease, dementia) are progressive and impact adversely on quality of life. Despite frailty being common in older age, and independently associated with important adverse outcomes, it is not routinely identified and coded in primary or secondary care in the manner which has become usual practice for other long-term conditions (Harrison et al., 2015). NHS England has, however, characterised frailty as a long-term condition that can be routinely identified and managed to improve a person's quality of life and wellbeing and to support them to live well for longer (NIHR Dissemination Centre, 2017).

Frailty has been associated with a number of adverse events. These include increased risk of cardiovascular disease, hypertension, cancer and death, even after adjusting for chronic conditions and disability. Surgery is a form of '**acute stress**', and frailty has been associated with higher complication rates and prolonged recovery (Velanovich et al., 2013). Researchers have demonstrated that even when individuals with acute and chronic medical conditions were excluded, 7 per cent of the population aged more than 65 years and 20 per cent of the population aged more than 80 years were frail (Ahmed et al., 2007).

Frailty is a heterogeneous and diverse condition, which might account for variations in definitions, phenotypic features and assessment methods. While it is not surprising that the mortality rate increases with age, it is striking that the increase is so simple – **the Gompertz law** for older humans shows that mortality increases exponentially with age (Gompertz, 1825). Lack of adaptive capacity can arise in many contexts, including any severe injury or widespread, systemic illness, but what intrigues researchers is the vulnerability that arises with age, even sometimes although not often in the absence of much frank illness (Song et al., 2010). This might be closely linked to intrinsic capacity, which I review in Chapter 7. Maintenance of health in old age is both a challenge and goal of the healthcare system. The proportion of people aged 65 and older is expected to increase worldwide in the coming decades. Reserve capacity decreases, and the risk of morbidity and frailty increases by ageing. There is a close link between ill health and frailty in older adults; a combination of multimorbidity, impairment of reserve and functional capacity, and dependency on others in daily activities is associated with frailty (Ebrahimi *et al.*, 2013).

Multimorbidity

Multimorbidity is a frequent occurrence, particularly in the elderly population, among whom prevalence was found to be greater than 60 per cent (Fortin *et al.*, 2012). Available data have shown negative consequences related to multimorbidity, including an increased risk of disability, frailty and decrease in quality of life, as well as associations with mortality (Nunes *et al.*, 2016).

It is important to understand the difference between frailty, long-term conditions and disability. There may be overlap between the management approaches for people with multimorbidity and those with frailty but these conditions are not identical. Multimorbidity is usually defined as the coexistence of two or more chronic diseases in the same individual (Radner *et al.*, 2014). It may be viewed as an evolution of the comorbidity concept, which refers to 'the existence or occurrence of any distinct additional entity during the clinical course of a patient who has the index disease under study' (Feinstein, 1970). It is readily evident that, as opposed to comorbidity, multimorbidity is a patient-centred entity, in which no index disease is predefined (Cesari *et al.*, 2017).

It is advised that one should consider assessing frailty in people with multimorbidity, but that one should be cautious about assessing frailty in a person who is acutely unwell, and one should not use a physical performance tool to assess frailty in a person who is acutely unwell ('Multimorbidity: clinical assessment and management', NICE guideline [NG56], published date: September 2016[6]). Multimorbidity is frequently complicated by an acute event that may lead to acute hospitalisation. Information on the prevalence of multimorbidity in acutely hospitalised older patients may be useful for everyday clinical practice to assist patients and their caregivers in decision making as well as inform them about the prognosis of the acute illness experienced in addition to their existing chronic diseases (Buurman *et al.*, 2016). Attempts to address the complex nature of frailty have often resulted in reformulation of the ageing processes in stochastic and multidimensional terms (Manton *et al.*, 1995). Of further clinical interest, frailty has been found to be at least in part *reversible* in some patients and the subject of preventive strategies. Potentially reversible risk factors for frailty, such as malnutrition, sarcopenia, cardiovascular changes and morbidity should be subjects for preventive and therapeutic strategies. Clearly, frailty is of major relevance especially in **but not limited to** geriatric medicine (Ritt *et al.*, 2016). Ageing and frailty are closely intertwined, but frail older adults are at a greater risk of accelerated decline in many aspects of function (Mitnitski *et al.*, 2017).

According to many specialists, frailty does not actually exist in the absence of chronic diseases. If no chronic comorbidity is known when frailty is diagnosed, sub-clinical or undiagnosed disease might therefore be present. Nevertheless, some characteristics of frailty apply for normal ageing, such as decreased physiological reserve and loss of complexity. It might therefore be very difficult or even impossible to distinguish frailty unambiguously from advanced stages of the ageing process (Sieber, 2017). Comorbidity should not be regarded as merely the sum of a number of diseases (or as the coexistence of multimorbidity) in the same patient. Because of the decision making that must follow, comorbidity is defined by establishing a hierarchy and relationships (e.g. in drug–drug interactions or in selecting priorities) existing in those situations. It is worth noting that Ford and Ford (2017) have recently questioned the term 'multimorbidity' for a number of reasons.

Health assets

Rotegård and colleagues (Rotegård *et al.*, 2010) have defined health assets as follows:

> Health assets are the repertoire of potentials – internal and external strength qualities in the individual's possession, both innate and acquired – that mobilize positive health behaviors and optimal health/wellness outcomes.

Basic ways to support a person living with frailty include looking after their health, e.g. looking after feet, mouth, eyes and hearing, getting vaccinations, taking medicines, personal hygiene, and attending to any changes in health proactively. Interventions should be ultimately made available which improve overall physical, mental and social functioning, using a goal-orientated rather than a disease-focused approach, taking account of individual needs and personal assets, *rather than deficits*.

An **assets-based approach** to health policy, research and practice aims to support individuals, communities and organisations to secure the skills and competencies that can maximise opportunities for health and wellbeing (Morgan and Ziglio, 2017). **This is all also about thinking differently** or 'reframing the narrative' – refocusing our questions to the 'glass half-full' of frailty. An assets-based approach concerns itself with identifying those protective factors that keep us well so that they can help offset the risks that inevitably people will face in their lives. This should not be directed only at members of silos of health and social care, as all people have a vested interested in preventing their patients from deteriorating health-wise.

Assets-based approaches also do not represent a model that stands in polar opposition to a deficit model, but instead they add value to a deficits approach. They operate alongside interventions targeted at reducing health risk behaviours (Morgan and Ziglio, 2007). The more health programmes are developed with and by local people, the more likely they are to be successful and sustainable (Popay *et al.*, 2007). Effective ways of involving people might include: a commitment by policy for long-term investment; openness to organisational and cultural change to understand what supports or inhibits community engagement; a willingness to share power fairly as appropriate, between statutory and community organisations; and the development of trust and respect among all those involved (Morgan and Hernán, 2013).

Potential strengths of an assets-based approach are shown in Box 1.1.

BOX 1.1 POTENTIAL STRENGTHS OF AN ASSET-BASED APPROACH

An asset-based approach:

- helps people to think positively about their circumstances;
- is realistic as it identifies what is already available;
- is inclusive and encourages equality and reciprocity needed for co-production;
- facilitates both independence and interdependencies;
- facilitates the valuing of others (what matters to people);
- provides a mechanism for the mobilisation of the assets;
- promotes the local population as a producer of health, rather than as a service user;
- encourages people to realise their ability to contribute to the development of health and wellbeing;
- facilitates the identification of a range of health promotion factors;
- helps to develop more sustainable initiatives;
- aims to empower people;
- helps to identify methods in which individuals can use their talents.

Based on Whiting et al., 2012, p. 27, Box 2.

Historically, approaches to the promotion of health have been based on an 'illness' model. The focus is mainly on risk factors for disease 'health deficits', rather than those associated with improving health status. While the presence of risk factors increases the likelihood of poor health, their absence does not necessarily increase the likelihood of good health (Hornby-Turner et al., 2017). This approach of identifying risk factors for disease is essential for understanding specific needs and priorities; however, it tends to define individuals in negative terms, and may overlook important positive factors which improve public health (Morgan and Ziglio, 2007). Indeed many participants in a recent qualitative study involving focus groups of community-dwelling older adults with diverse age and frailty status revealed that information about how to treat or prevent frailty and the risks associated with being frail can be conveyed without necessarily using the specific term 'frail', which they perceived to have a negative connotation (Schoenborn et al., 2018).

The core of the health concept is **wellness**, a quality that must be appraised and assessed from the patient's perspective and experience (Moore and Huerena, 2005). Wellness is based on the promotion and maintenance of health and capacities for living rather than on healing of poor health and solving problems (Carlson, 2003).

Asset-based approaches have a different starting point to traditional health and care services. Fundamentally, they ask the question 'what makes us healthy?', rather than the deficit-based question 'what makes us ill?' Asset-based approaches are not a replacement for investing in service improvement or attempting to address the structural causes of health inequalities. Fortunately, the detrimental effects of frailty are not deterministic and can be buffered against by high spirituality (Kirby *et al.*, 2004) and sufficient financial resources (Hubbard *et al.*, 2014).

A first major publication produced by the Rockwood group had indeed elaborated a model of frailty that stresses 'a complex interplay of assets and deficits, "medical" and "social", that maintain health or threaten independence' (Rockwood *et al.*, 1994, pp. 490–1). This was based explicitly on a notion of balance, developing the work of John Brocklehurst, a second-generation pioneer in geriatric medicine, between positive and negative factors in everyday life.

Social determinants of frailty and 'reframing the narrative'

Many non-communicable diseases including frailty that cause the greatest burden on health in England are preventable, caused by unhealthy behaviours such as smoking, and eating and drinking to excess. Promoting healthy lifestyles and empowering individuals to make healthy choices is central to Public Health England's work to tackle long-term, chronic diseases, including frailty, and reduce preventable deaths and disability. Reducing inequalities is a central aim of this. Impairment and personal strengths are closely connected. Current research shows that psychological and social resources correspond to physiological resilience (Meeks *et al.*, 2016) and that active participation in the treatment process (based on the personal strengths of the individual) is fundamental for the process of recovery (Kessing *et al.*, 2014; Steunenberg *et al.*, 2007). However, it seems that the mere availability of close social ties, such as family members, does not simply facilitate resilience (Sherman *et al.*, 2013). Schlotfeldt refers to experience as both impeding and enhancing a person's attainment of optimal health (Glazer and Pressler, 1989).

The **Marmot Review** had identified six policy recommendations to reduce health inequalities, including creating 'healthy and sustainable places and communities'. The links that connect people within communities provide a source of resilience, access to support, opportunities for participation and added control over their lives; they have the potential to 'contribute to psychosocial wellbeing and as a result to other health outcomes' (Marmot, 2010). Connectedness, networks, trust, reciprocity and feelings of belonging are the 'social glue' that binds people and places together, and are important for promoting both health and wellbeing.

In persons who are frail, it has been found that low psychosocial resources led to additional days of inpatient treatment and re-hospitalisation (Hoogendijk *et al.*,

2014). On the other hand, in depressive individuals, self-efficacy has been shown to have a mediating effect on treatment adherence and outcome (Bisschop *et al.*, 2004). Dent and Hoogendijk (2014) also found that psychosocial factors conferred protection against adverse outcomes for frail adults in a hospitalised cohort. In contrast, this was not found in a community cohort which also included frail older adults and examined mortality and functional decline (Hoogendijk *et al.*, 2014). *If* frailty is a consequence of cumulative decline in multiple physiological systems, information about its aetiology might come from studying determinants of frailty decades before its onset. In a recent study, involving 876 members of the Lothian Birth Cohort, significant associations between lower intelligence and greater socio-economic disadvantage in childhood – as indicated by father's social class – and increased risk of frailty at age 70 were found to be attenuated, and no longer significant after adjustments for the potential mediating factors, educational attainment, attained social class and health behaviours in adulthood (Gale *et al.*, 2016).

Salutogenesis

'**Salutogenesis**' describes an approach focusing on factors that support wellbeing and health rather than factors that cause disease (Lindstrom and Eriksson, 2005).

The development of the concept of health assets, particularly within a public health arena, has been influenced by salutogenesis (Antonovsky, 1987, 1996). An assets-based model of health fits well with salutogenesis since it emphasises the positive capacity of communities to promote the health of its members (Kawachi, 2010). Antonovsky coined the term 'salutogenesis', meaning the 'origins of health' (Antonovsky, 1996, p. 13). Antonovsky (1996, p. 11) thought of salutogenesis as a more appropriate health promotion approach than the more traditional 'disease orientation' focus as it concentrates on 'moving people in the direction of the health end of a healthy/disease continuum'. Health promotion aims to create equitable conditions for health for the entire population (World Health Organization, 1986). However, one still has to be mindful that vulnerable groups may have limited opportunities to access and benefit from health promotion initiatives. For example, Baum (2000) finds that participation in local groupings is more likely to take place among the more privileged members of society. The power of participation to catalyse a process of social transformation and more inclusive democracies can therefore be easily undermined by the lack of representation from all groups (Hindhede and Aagaard-Hansen, 2017).

Community assets

It is important to be able to support people living with frailty and those important to them to access local community groups and services and to understand the benefit this could bring, and also to consider the support network of friends, family and others around an individual (referred to as a 'caring network'), which may extend beyond immediate family and friends.

Involving people who are frail is important.

> A crucial aspect of any asset-based approach is the involvement of people in decisions and processes that have the potential to impact upon them. Without this participation, there is a danger that there will not be true representation of the assets that are most important for that particular person or group – this could mean that policy makers will continue to drive the health and well-being agenda forward without the support of those who really matter. Practitioners should think carefully about the circumstances in which an asset-based approach would be used, as it may not be appropriate for every situation.
>
> *(Whiting* et al., *2012)*

Policy makers across the world are becoming increasingly interested in improving health and wellbeing by creating a more inclusive community-based society. Newspaper and magazine articles, television advertisements, posters and even books suggest that to live healthily and happily well into advanced old age an individual must be a 'smart consumer', who makes informed choices about purchasing and utilising appropriate products, from 'organic foods to to gym memberships' for example (Chivers, 2003). Foot and Hopkins (2010) have argued that community assets can achieve a number of goals, including (1) providing new ways of challenging health inequalities; (2) valuing resilience; (3) strengthening community networks; and (4) recognising local expertise.

Social resources, such as **social capital**, have been linked to the absence of loneliness among the general population (Islam *et al.*, 2006; Kim *et al.*, 2007) as well as among older people (Routasalo *et al.*, 2009). The social networks within communities create 'social capital', resources such as support, reciprocity through volunteering networks and links which bridge divides of power, status, knowledge and access. This in real life means having a social life and accessing community resources. The quality and quantity of complex social relationships with family, friends and social networks have been shown to affect morbidity and mortality. Nevertheless, there is evidence to suggest that people with stronger social networks tend to be stronger, healthier and happier (Marmot, 2010). Critical to this is the social contact and social support that fosters greater self-confidence and reduces isolation in communities: 'individuals need communities and communities need engaged citizens to survive' (Friedli and Parsonage, 2009, p. 15). A wider goal is to facilitate augmentation of social networks to promote communication between aged/frail people, their relatives, caregivers and health professionals.[7] Care partners may be reluctant to accept help, because they feel they should be able to handle everything themselves; but they should get used to saying yes to 'offers of help' and learning how to ask for help.[8]

It is also worth noting that being part of a community can make a difference to the perception of an interaction with the health and social care services.

> With a notable frequency, patients and relatives describe the relationships they had with staff and each other as the key feature of their acute care

experience. For patients, a 'connected' and reciprocal relationship with staff provided reassurance that staff recognised and would meet all their needs for treatment and care, and that they were safe, legitimate as a patient in receipt of acute care and significant as a human being that matters to others. Maintaining connections with family and social networks also helped patients feel supported and connected.

(Bridges et al., 2010, p. 93)

In later work, Kretzmann and McKnight (1993) introduced the '**Asset Based Community Development**' (ABCD), a system in which a community increases the health and wellbeing of its population using activities, skills and assets of (lower-income) people and neighbourhoods. Using an ABCD approach enables communities to build on what assets they have to gain what they need and make improvements to their community, and thereby improve individual and community-level health and wellbeing.

Communities that are more 'cohesive', characterised by strong social bonds and ties, have been shown to be more likely to maintain and sustain health even in the face of disadvantage (Harrison *et al.*, 2004; Magis, 2010; Morgan and Ziglio, 2007). A meta-analysis of 148 studies investigating the association between social relationships and mortality indicated that individuals with adequate social relationships have a 50 per cent greater likelihood of survival compared with those with poor or insufficient relationships (Holt-Lunstad *et al.*, 2010). The authors hypothesised that this may function through a stress-buffering mechanism or behavioural modelling, within social networks. Community intervention approaches hold widespread appeal in health promotion and as such many have originated in response to the guiding principles of the Ottawa Charter (World Health Organization, 1986). The **Ottawa Charter** declares that health promotion is 'the process of enabling people to increase control over their health and its determinants, and thereby improve their health. It moves beyond a focus on individual behaviour towards a wide range of social and environmental interventions'.

Capabilities refer to the specific functionings that are feasible for an individual to choose to achieve. An individual has a certain capability if the individual is able to achieve the corresponding functioning, given his or her available personal, material, social, institutional and legal resources. An individual's capabilities, then, are a function of the real options he or she has available (Murphy and Gardoni, 2006). A capabilities approach, in broad terms, is a new theoretical paradigm that conceptualises social justice in terms of equality of opportunities for the individuals to be and do what they value (Silva and Howe, 2012).

The actual identity of frailty

The framing of what frailty actually is cannot be easily assumed. A qualitative study of older people aged 66–98 years found that 'most participants actively resented the identity', even those who could be classified as frail using objective criteria

(Warmoth *et al.*, 2016). The diagnosis of frailty also appears to have a subjective dimension. Qualitative research shows that being diagnosed as frail by others can contribute to the development of a frailty identity that leads to behavioural changes, including a lesser participation in social activities (Warmoth *et al.*, 2016). That is why it is so important to act on day-to-day interactions with people to encourage changes in behaviour that will have a positive impact on the health and wellbeing of individuals, communities and populations, i.e. 'Making every contact count'.[9] The well-known '**frailty phenotype**' introduced by Fried and colleagues (2001) which classifies people into categories of robust, pre-frail or frail, fits within this physiological approach to frailty. It is postulated that five indicators – weight loss, exhaustion, slow walking speed, low grip strength and low level of physical activity – are related to each other in the frailty phenotype.

The term 'pre-frailty' is sometimes used to describe patients who may be at risk for frailty. Although no exact definition exists, these patients typically have some components of a frailty measure but not enough to meet the defined frailty cut-off. Similar to frailty, although prefrailty is often thought of as an age-related condition, it is critical to recognise that it also can exist in young patients. Pre-frailty is commonly assessed using the Fried phenotype (presence of one–two of the following: slow gait speed, weakness, low energy, unintentional weight loss and low physical activity) (Fried *et al.*, 2001). Though less vulnerable than frail older adults, pre-frail people are at higher risk than robust adults of greater frailty, hospitalisation, falls, worsening disability and mortality (Fried *et al.*, 2001). Older people with mild or pre-frailty are more likely to transition back to a robust state than those who are frail, and so health promotion represents an important opportunity to prevent decline and dependence, and to potentially make gains in health and reductions in disability and need for care (Frost *et al.*, 2017). But it is more likely using a dimensional approach that pre-frailty reflects a state of deficits and assets which have not manifest yet as overt symptoms across a broad range of phenotypes.

Introduction to assessing frailty

Health and social care professionals have ways of assessing frailty which can help in planning appropriate care and support. Demographic changes have led to an increase in the number of elderly frail persons and, consequently, systematic geriatric assessment is more important than ever. Detection or identification of frailty, most agree, is a crucial first step in treating frailty in older people. It is, however, vital to be aware of the experience of a person with frailty and their family and care partners, and be able to communicate with sensitivity about the assessment of frailty and related implications. Various operational definitions have been proposed to assess the frailty condition among older individuals. An online survey was sent to national geriatric societies affiliated to the European Union Geriatric Medicine Society (EUGMS) and to members of the European Society for Clinical and Economic Aspects of Osteoporosis, Osteoarthritis and Musculoskeletal Diseases (Bruyère *et al.*, 2017). A substantial proportion of clinicians (64.9 per cent) diagnose frailty using more than one instrument. The most widely used tool was the gait speed test, adopted by 43.8 per cent of the clinicians, followed by clinical frailty scale (34.3 per cent), the SPPB (short physical performance battery) test (30.2 per cent), the frailty phenotype (26.8 per cent) and the frailty index (16.8 per cent).

It has been shown that tools at these ends of the spectrum are for different purposes: as an indicator of population healthy ageing or as a tool for clinical use (Woo et al., 2012).

A range of simple tests for identifying frailty is available. Slow walking speed (less than 0.8 m/s or taking more than 5 seconds to walk 4 m); the PRISMA 7 questionnaire and the timed–up–and–go test (with a cut–off score of 10 seconds) had very good sensitivity but only moderate specificity for identifying frailty. This means that there are many fitter older people who will have a positive test result (false positives).

- **Gait speed**: taking more than 5 seconds to cover 4 m. Gait speed is usually measured in m/s and has been recorded over distances ranging from 2.4 to 6 m in research studies.[10]
- **Timed up-and-go test** (TUGT): taking more than 10 seconds to get up from a chair, walk 3 m, turn around and sit down (Podsiadlo and Richardson, 1991). This clinical test, developed in a medical setting, asks subjects to wear their regular footwear and use their customary walking aid (none, cane, walker). No physical assistance is given. The TUG is well known and widely used where the clinical goal is to get an accurate objective assessment of balance, and the scoring system is easy to use and provides a clinically useful indicator of falls risk for ambulatory older adults.
- The **PRISMA 7** (Program of Research to Integrate Services for the Maintenance of Autonomy) is a seven–item, self–completion questionnaire.[11] The questions are shown in Box 1.2.

BOX 1.2 PRISMA 7 QUESTIONS

1 Are you more than 85 years?
2 Male?
3 In general do you have any health problems that require you to limit your activities?
4 Do you need someone to help you on a regular basis?
5 In general do you have any health problems that require you to stay at home?
6 In case of need can you count on someone close to you?
7 Do you regularly use a stick, walker or wheelchair to get about?

Raîche et al., 2007

A brief clinical assessment would help exclude some false positives (e.g. fit older people with isolated knee arthritis causing slow gait speed), for example. Various fuller tools have been proposed to 'measure frailty'. Table 1.2 shows *some* of them.

It is important to explain the need for an assessment of frailty with sensitivity and in ways that are appropriate and acceptable to the person. There is currently a need

TABLE 1.2 Description of the tools commonly used to assess frailty

Clinical frailty scale	This is based on a clinical evaluation in the domains of mobility, energy, physical activity and function, using descriptors and figures to stratify elderly adults according to their level of vulnerability.
SPPB	The short physical performance battery (SPPB) test is composed of three separate tests: balance, 4-metre gait speed and chair stand test.
Frailty phenotype	This is a deficit across five domains. Thus, phenotype of frailty was identified by the presence of three or more of the following components: shrinking, weakness, poor endurance and energy, slowness and a low level of physical activity.
Frailty index	This is expressed as a ratio of deficits present to the total number of deficits considered. Frailty index includes 40 variables and the calculation was performed on the maximum number of deficits collected. Thus, participants were considered as frail when the ratio of deficits present to the total number of deficits considered was 0.25 (i.e. lowest quartile) or more.
Gerontopole frailty screening tool	This is an eight-item questionnaire intended to help general practitioners identify frailty in community-dwelling persons 65 years or older without functional disability or current acute disease. The first six questions evaluate the patient's status whereas the last two assess the general practitioner's personal view about the frailty status of the individual and the patient's willingness to be referred to the Frailty Clinical for further evaluation.
SHARE frailty instrument	Using the five SHARE frailty variables (fatigue, loss of appetite, grip strength, functional difficulties and physical activity), D-factor scores (DFS) are determined using the SHARE-FI formula.
Groningen frailty indicator	This consists of 15 self-report items and screens for loss of functions and resources in four domains: physical, cognitive, social and psychological. Scores range from 0 (not frail) to 15 (very frail). A GFI score of 4 or higher is regarded as frail.

Source: based on Bruyère *et al.*, 2017, p. 907, Table 1.

for additional evidence to guide decision making for the care of frail patients, since frail persons are frequently excluded from studies, the differential impact of frailty is often not examined in clinical trials and few large-scale clinical trials examining frail cohorts have been conducted (Shears *et al.*, 2017). Randomised control trials published to date have used a diverse range of definitions of frailty, as well as a variety of outcome measures.

The 'frailty index'

Over the past few decades, many screening tools have been developed to identify frailty in older people. Despite the importance of multiple domains, only a small number of instruments take different frailty domains into account. The **frailty index** (FI) is possibly the second most widely applied instrument and is based on a deficit accumulation approach (Rockwood and Mitnitski, 2007; Rockwood *et al.*, 2004; Mitnitski *et al.*, 2001). A count is taken of deficits which are a collection of symptoms, signs, diseases, disabilities or test abnormalities. Selected deficits should be associated with poorer health status, should increase with age but not saturate too early, must as a group cover a range of systems, and must be the same for a group of people followed serially (Searle *et al.*, 2008). An increasing number of deficits raise the likelihood of being frail. It is expressed as the ratio of actual number of deficits to total possible number of deficits and is therefore a scalar measure ranging from 0 to 1. Perhaps most intriguingly, it appears that, at least by the age of 70, vulnerability to adverse health outcomes can be predicted by considering a broad range of data, including self-reported information (Rockwood *et al.*, 2006).

A frailty index can be generated from almost any set of health-related variables, as long as a few criteria are met. The criteria for an item to be considered as a deficit are that the item needs to be acquired, age-associated and associated with an adverse outcome, and should not saturate too early. An example would be nocturia in men. Although nocturia is age associated, interrupts sleep, and is a deficit, the problem is common, typically seen in more than 90 per cent of men older than 75 years (Rockwood and Mitninski, 2011). There is a growing literature on the interaction between comorbid illness and frailty, which suggests that rather than taking these concepts separately, frailty can be viewed, at least in part, as one result of the accu-mulation of the burden of chronic, multiple comorbid illness over time (Sales, 2009). Whilst the trajectory of ageing can differ among older people, there is general agreement that ageing is associated with an accumulation of cellular damage (Soysal *et al.*, 2017).

The index is actually very elegant. A consistent thread in the Rockwood research is how the index reflects the need of older-age epidemiology to reflect the com-plexity of interacting conditions.

For example,

> Such considerations also inform our approach, but with a different take that, in our view, has consequences for both dementia epidemiology and potentially

for management. Instead of picking out factors that only individually are statistically significant, and then seeing whether they survive multivariable modeling, we were struck by the fact that different subsets of variables can give comparable predictions.

(Song, Mitnitski and Rockwood, 2014)

The health of individuals is highly heterogeneous, as is the rate at which they age. The accumulation of deficits definition of frailty, often termed the frailty index, proposes that frailty is a non-specific age-associated vulnerability that is reflected in an accumulation of medical, social and functional deficits and that can be measured by counting an individual's health problems or deficits (Rockwood and Mitnitski, 2007). Changes in the frailty index characterise the rate of individual ageing, it is argued. The behaviour of the FI is highly characteristic: it shows an age specific, non-linear increase, higher values in females, strong associations with adverse outcomes (e.g. mortality) (Mitniski *et al.*, 2013). Not everyone accumulates deficits at the same rate, nor do they accumulate the same deficits. Deficits can be summarised in a frailty index, which counts the proportion that is present in a given individual and, interestingly, the index seems to converge to a maximum level beyond which the disruption of homeostasis has catastrophic consequences for the individual, thus marking a salient health transition towards death (Rockwood and Mitnitski, 2006).

The application of a frailty index may have added value for longitudinal studies in older populations. For these studies, a valid and sensitive frailty instrument is important so that the impact of frailty on various outcomes can be studied, as can its trajectory. In addition, it is imperative to apply the frailty index in different studies, to be able to compare its characteristics across different countries and settings (Hoogendijk *et al.*, 2017). But it could be argued that the longitudinal design of 'intrinsic capacity' strongly promotes the transition from a reactive towards a preventive model of medicine. (I discuss 'intrinsic capacity' in Chapter 8.)

Whether reversing deficits changes prognosis, or whether, in samples of people who present with acute illness, there are also pragmatic limits to deficit accumulation, are interesting questions that are motivating further research (Rockwood and Mitnitski, 2006). Also absent from the accumulation of deficits index is any guide to the impact of the 'temporal ordering' of these deficits. Temporal ordering is a feature of cascade theories of ageing in which accumulation of deficits occur in a general sequence, potentially leading to an acceleration of decline once a threshold is reached (Anstey and Dixon, 2014).

The frailty phenotype

Frailty phenotypes and indices are complementary not competing views. The **frailty phenotype** (FP) defined by Fried and colleagues also presents some limitations for clinical practice and research purposes. First, several biological mechanisms of the clinical syndrome (obesity, inflammation, hormonal changes, low muscle strength, sarcopenia, insulin resistance, sedentariness, poor cardiovascular balance and so on) seem to be interdependent, generating a continuous gradient of multi-systemic biological dysfunction from vigorous to the most vulnerable individual. The FP was first described by Fried and colleagues (2001) in the Cardiovascular Health Study, in the United States, and focuses on five traits associated with being frail, and that normally become more pronounced with age.

Recent findings with the frailty phenotype indicate that the first longitudinal data that raise the possibility that the higher prevalence of frailty observed in ethnic minority groups using the original frailty phenotype may be related in large part to ethnic differences in body composition, because they disappear when frailty criteria are standardised to body composition characteristics. Thus, this higher prevalence may not represent a truly higher vulnerability to stress and functional decline (Alonso Bouzón *et al.*, 2017).

A problem persists that many people refer to frailty when talking about different things. It's like concentrating on the trunk rather than the tail of an elephant. In a further 'twist' of definitions, a post by the British Geriatrics Society[12] explains that occasionally frailty means that individuals can present with what appears to be a straight-forward symptom masking a more serious or complex underlying medical problem.

This approach gives rise to the concept of 'frailty syndromes' (previously known as the 'geriatric giants') and should encourage a search for the underlying cause:

1   falls (e.g. collapse, legs gave way, 'found lying on floor');
2   immobility (e.g. sudden change in mobility, 'gone off legs', 'stuck in toilet');
3   delirium (e.g. acute confusion, 'muddledness', sudden worsening of confusion in someone with previous dementia or known memory loss);
4   incontinence (e.g. change in continence – new onset or worsening of urine or faecal incontinence);
5   susceptibility to side effects of medication (e.g. confusion with codeine, hypo-tension with antidepressants).

Frailty syndromes may indeed be a first presentation of frailty, and it is important to have a basic idea of what could be acute presentations of these frailty syndromes, or to prevent them happening in the first place.

Definition of health

A burning issue is whether frailty is a state of health, illness or disease, or 'all of the above'? Several dimensions of health can be identified in the social domain, includ-ing people's capacity to fulfil their potential and obligations, the ability to manage their life with some degree of independence despite a medical condition, and the ability to participate in social activities including work. Health in this domain can be regarded as a dynamic balance between opportunities and limitations, shifting through life and affected by external conditions such as social and environmental challenges (Huffman *et al.*, 2016). Complex dynamical systems theory hypothesises that any complex system, like a human being, is permanently subject to natural perturbations from the environment (Gijzel *et al.*, 2017).

The concept of health has changed in accordance with the knowledge, beliefs and values of each historical and socio-cultural period. Frailty holds an ambiguous identity as a state of both health, illness and disease. The traditional approach that equates health with absence of disease and focuses on the individual has progressed toward a more dynamic, multicomponent, positive, holistic and collective definition that considers health a universal human right (Pons-Vigués *et al.*, 2017). The current WHO definition of health, formulated in 1948, describes health as 'a state of complete physical, mental and social well-being and not merely the absence of disease or infirmity'.[13] At that time, this formulation was ground-breaking because of its breadth and ambition. It overcame the negative definition of health as absence of disease and included the physical, mental, and social domains. Most criticism of the WHO definition concerns the absoluteness of the word 'complete' in relation to wellbeing. The first problem is that it unintentionally contributes to the overall medicalisation of society (Huber *et al.*, 2011). The time, some believe, has come to abandon '**the disease entity**' as the focus of medical care. The current approach of medical care that is centred on the diagnosis and treatment of individual diseases is at best out of date and at worst harmful; it seems that a primary focus on disease may inadvertently lead to under-treatment, over-treatment or mis-treatment (Tinetti and Fried, 2004).

Several dimensions of health can be identified in the social domain. Health in this domain can be regarded as a dynamic balance between opportunities and limitations, shifting through life and affected by external conditions such as social and environmental challenges (Huber *et al.*, 2011). The classic WHO definition of health as complete wellbeing has recently been challenged. Whilst health is not simply an absence of illness, it is clear that promoting health in people living with frailty needs alertness about treating illness. For example, it is crucial to be able to support a person living with frailty in looking after their health, e.g. looking after feet, mouth, eyes and hearing, getting vaccinations, taking medicines, personal hygiene or attending to any changes in health proactively.

An introduction to resilience

Frailty, stress and resilience are three words which now keep regular company together (Conti and Conti, 2010). Ageing presents itself to a greater or lesser degree from 'successful' ageing to 'pathological' ageing depending on the reserve functions of the different physiological systems, their resilience and the consequent appearance of disease (Fulop *et al.*, 2010). A desire to know who adapts to adversity more effectively (and why) has led to ongoing interest in the capacity for resilience – the ability to overcome or bounce back from adversity, with a suggestion that resilience is available to everybody (Bonanno *et al.*, 2006).

Resilience, or 'the ability to adapt positively to adversity', is a psychological construct that has been examined in relation to an individual's response to cancer (Aspinwall and MacNamara, 2005), traumatic stress (Charney, 2004) and other challenging life circumstances. While not a fully realised construct, resilience and other similar adaptive processes are posited to be important to successful ageing (Baltes, 1997; Hardy *et al.*, 2002; Schulz and Heckhausen, 1996). Some view resilience as a response to a specific event, such as a trauma, whereas others treat resilience as a stable coping style (Luthar *et al.*, 2000). Coping with impairment implies managing the demands created by stressful events. Coping resources play an important role in this process (Lazarus and Folkman, 1984; Taylor and Stanton, 2007). Population ageing is a key social challenge of our time. As governments strive to reduce the costs of elder care in the context of a decreasing population of younger people entering the workforce, successful ageing has become a popular concept that refers to simultaneous reduction of disease and disability, maintenance of cognitive and physical functioning, and active social engagement throughout the life-course and into later life (Rowe and Kahn, 1998).

The debate about 'how much people go back to normal after a shock' will be critical here. Varadhan *et al.* (2018) specifically propose that 'resilience' ought to be defined as the ability of a system to recover from a perturbation of sufficiently large magnitude (a stressor) that the system is pushed into a state far from its original equilibrium state, ultimately retaining essential identity and function. The authors distinguish resilience subtly from 'robustness', further defined, where a robust system can move far away from its original equilibrium into a new state of equilibrium without any discernible change in its performance.

Coping strategies

Coping strategies are essential to minimise the impact of stress and determine the degree of resilience or susceptibility. Coping is active when an individual tries to deal with a challenge, faces fears, participates in problem solving and seeks social support (Franklin *et al.*, 2012). It also engages optimism and positive reassessment of aversive experiences that can produce long-term resilience. In contrast, passive coping involves denial, avoidance of conflicts, suppression of emotions, and behavioural disengagement. Coping style varies between individuals and situations and influences how the neuroendocrine and neuroimmunological systems are activated in response to stress (Zozulya *et al.*, 2008).

Vulnerability

Recent work has proposed a helpful taxonomy distinguishing three sources and two states of vulnerability. Considered in terms of its sources, vulnerability may be inherent, situational or pathogenic (e.g. Rogers *et al.*, 2012).

- *Inherent vulnerability* is the form of vulnerability 'intrinsic to the human condition'.

- *Situational vulnerability* is context-specific: it is caused or exacerbated by the temporary or enduring conditions in which agents find themselves.
- *Pathogenic vulnerability* refers to sources of vulnerability that arise from the exacerbation or compounding of existing vulnerability.

Community capability and social vulnerability

Resilience has much to do with community capability and social vulnerability. 'Community capability' is the combined influence of a community's social systems and collective resources that can be applied to address community problems and broaden community opportunities. Norton and colleagues (2002) define it as 'a set of dynamic community traits, resources, and associational patterns that can be brought to bear for community building and community health improvement' (Norton *et al.*, 2002).

Social vulnerability can be a risk factor for poor health outcomes and an important aspect to consider for healthcare provision and planning (Wallace *et al.*, 2015). Shankar and colleagues found significant interaction effects of isolation and loneliness, indicating the need to study the effects of these social factors simultaneously (Shankar *et al.*, 2013). It appears possible to compile series of social factors and found that an accumulation of social deficits is predictive of future cognitive transitions, warranting further research attention to potential interventions that may lessen the burden of social vulnerability in older adults (Armstrong *et al.*, 2015). Since the concept of social frailty comprises a complex, dynamic interaction of resources, activities and abilities for fulfilling the social needs of individual older adults, an index to measure social frailty could provide insights into their specific healthcare and social care needs (Bunt *et al.*, 2017). The **Social Vulnerability Index** (SVI) was developed for this purpose, providing a holistic quantification of social vulnerability among older people and appearing to be a valid measure (e.g. Wallace *et al.*, 2015; Andrew and Rockwood, 2010). The SVI is a multifactorial and multilevel index that consists of items that reflect particular aspects of a person's social circumstances. Rather than focusing on one social dimension, the index includes a broad range of social factors, thereby creating a holistic measure of social vulnerability.

Vulnerability can also be approached from the viewpoint of the molecular level. Glucocorticoids play an important role in both the onset and the termination of the stress–response. Recent data from neurophysiological and behavioural studies suggest that glucocorticoids actually can enhance in the 'limbic brain' the initial stress reactions, which they prevent subsequently from overshooting.

Prolonged stress and vulnerability

Prolonged stress induces neuroimmune and neuroendocrine responses, and individual differences in these responses likely shape behavioural vulnerability and resilience. In some individuals, overactive, unresolved stress responses may increase stress vulnerability and ultimately the development of mood disorders (Charney, 2004). However, most individuals mount fairly adaptive coping mechanisms that promote resilience in the face of stress (Ménard *et al.*, 2017). The theoretical literature on frailty has hypothesised that changes in the regulatory systems involved in the maintenance of homeostasis may well be subtle and undetectable in the absence of external stressors (Buchner and Wagner, 1992). Therefore 'resilience' is a characteristic most observable in situations where an external stimulus induces measurable changes in the physiological system under a particular study.

The effects of stress can be prolonged as shown in Figure 1.1.

Frailty may be considered to reflect an intermediate, but distinct state between these two extremes, where a certain reversibility of pathological processes may still exist (Bortz, 2002). Vulnerability may be defined as an internal risk factor of the subject or system that is exposed to a hazard and corresponds to its intrinsic predisposition to be affected, or to be susceptible to damage. In other words, vulnerability represents the 'physical, economic, political or social susceptibility or predisposition of a community to damage in the case of a destabilising phenomenon of natural or anthropogenic origin' (Cardona, 2004, p. 37).

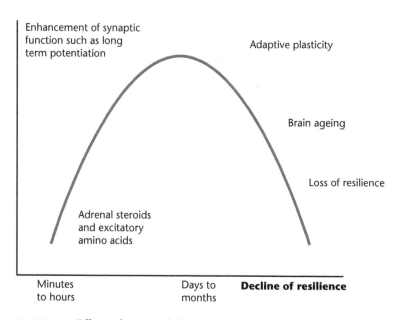

FIGURE 1.1   Effects of acute and chronic stress

Source: based on Figure 1, p. 1353 of McEwen BS, Bowles NP, Gray JD, Hill MN, Hunter RG, Karatsoreos IN, Nasca C. (2015). Mechanisms of stress in the brain. *Nat Neurosci*. October; 18(10): 1353–63. doi:10.1038/nn.4086. Epub 2015 September 25.

Note
These effects follow an inverted U-shaped curve in dose and time. The timeline shows how acute and chronic stress and ageing interact with the intensity and duration of stressor.

Stigma, prejudice and labelling, and engagement with personal care and support plans

I cannot apologise for wishing to identify stigma as a major issue for people given a label of 'frailty' in such a way that *does not disempower them individually*. Whilst one can argue until the cows come home whether a label of frailty is as stigmatising as that of genital herpes, the impact of 'otherness' is important. Effective communication creates opportunities to identify goals and actions for supported self-care, and to build the necessary motivation and confidence to carry out the necessary changes, but in truth this is potentially compromised by stigma.

Stigma is a mark separating individuals from one another based on a socially conferred judgment that some persons or groups are tainted and 'less than'. Stigma often leads to negative beliefs (e.g. stereotypes), the endorsement of those negative stereotypes as real (e.g. prejudice) and a desire to avoid or exclude persons who hold stigmatised statuses (Pescosolido *et al.*, 2008). The degree to which any condition can be considered to be stigmatising depends upon a number of factors, including whether the individual is viewed as responsible for the condition, the impact of the illness on others and the outward appearance or ability change associated with the condition (Reingold and Krishnan, 2001). Some statements about 'stigma' and 'deviance' are shown in Box 1.3 below.

BOX 1.3 CONCEPTUAL DISTINCTIONS FOR STIGMA AND DEVIANCE

Stigma: an ontological deficit, reflecting infringements against norms of shame
Deviance: a moral deficit, reflecting infringements against norms of blame
Enacted: discrimination by others on grounds of 'being imperfect'
Felt: internalised sense of shame and immobilising anticipation of enacted stigma

Based on Scambler, 2009, p. 451, Box 2.

Stigma is a pervasive influence on disease and responses of nations, communities, families and individuals to illness (Keusch *et al.*, 2006). Stigma occurs when elements of labelling, stereotyping, cognitive separation into categories of 'us' and 'them', status loss and discrimination co-occur in a power situation that allows these components to unfold (Link and Phelan, 2001). Whenever you think of 'othering', you should think of who is doing the othering and why. The denial of full humanness to others, and the cruelty and suffering that accompany it, is an all-too familiar phenomenon. However, arguably the concept of '**dehumanisation**' has rarely received systematic theoretical analysis (Haslam, 2006). Self-management can include physical activity, healthy diet, smoking cessation, vaccination and moderation of alcohol consumption (Sabia *et al.*, 2012). Additionally, engaging frail older adults in care planning will ensure that their goals and values are respected (You *et al.*, 2014), and might, for example, be shared with interested stakeholders, such as ambulance or other acute care professionals.

Integrated personalised care and support is therefore pivotal.

> For health, care and support to be 'integrated', it must be person-centred, coordinated, and tailored to the needs and preferences of the individual, their carer and family. It means moving away from episodic care to a more holistic approach to health, care and support needs, that puts the needs and experience of people at the centre of how services are organised and delivered.
>
> *(NHS England, Integrated care and support)*[14]

As such, it is unclear whether healthcare providers' understanding of frailty aligns with the experiences of well and frail older adults. Understanding these diverse perspectives is an integral step to rectifying potential misalignments and improving the appropriateness and effectiveness of health service provision for older adults along the frailty spectrum (Archibald *et al.*, 2017). Stigma is entirely relevant to all of this and is defined as 'typically a social process, experienced or anticipated, characterized by exclusion, rejection, blame or devaluation that results from experience, perception or reasonable anticipation of an adverse social judgement about a person or group' (Scambler, 2009, p. 441). Stigma often leads to negative beliefs (i.e. stereotypes), the endorsement of those negative stereotypes as real (i.e. prejudice) and a desire to avoid or exclude persons who hold stigmatised statuses (i.e. discrimination, Corrigan *et al.*, 2016; Link and Phelan, 2001). Levy (2009) points out that ageing stereotypes may influence older adults' wellbeing; as such, it may be useful to learn whether and how stories about successful ageing in various contexts inspire older adults to make better choices in their lives or cause resentment and disappointment because they shine a light on their own inadequate choices. This is of direct relevance to the identity and perception of frailty. The stigma surrounding frailty in particular is interesting from the vantage point of the view that 'we all recognise stigma when we see it'. As discussed in Green (2009), hiding the outward 'signs' of disease may help to conceal the impact of disease, but it is worth examining critically the traditional discourses of 'loss of self' due to marginalisation and social exclusion as, sometimes even, 'hero status' is achieved in the mass media.

All of this requires a far greater scrutiny of the label of 'frailty', and how it is perceived by others. Recently published results from a qualitative study involving 'focus groups' of community-dwelling older adults with diverse age and frailty status suggest that negative perceptions around the term 'frail' may be a barrier to the clinical application of frailty as a syndrome (Schoenborn *et al.*, 2018). The authors suggested that a different term to represent the concept of physical vulnerability may be preferable to patients and should be examined in future studies.

Carers and care planning

Carers are integral. According to the Carers Trust, a carer is 'anyone who cares, unpaid, for a friend or family member who due to illness, disability, a mental health problem or an addiction cannot cope without their support'.[15] The environment of care can have a profound impact on caregiving experiences of families caring for loved ones with a life-limiting illness, but care tends often to be delivered through disease-specific specialty clinics that are shaped by the illness trajectory (Penrod *et al.*, 2012). It is of fundamental interest whether personalised care planning (PCP) for older people with frailty improves quality of life and reduces health and social care resource use later, for example at 12 months. One aim of a recent NIHR grant is to optimise the Age UK integrated care service to deliver PCP for older people with frailty.[16]

Two important research outputs are identification of the target population for PCP in frailty, using the eFI (electronic frailty index) as a well-validated and widely available tool, and the development of a suitably optimised PCP intervention, including a common framework for routine NHS delivery. The PCP documents a plan to optimise and maintain health and function, an escalation plan advising when the patient/carer might need to seek further advice, an urgent care plan and, when appropriate, an end of life care plan. In an emergency situation, the presentation of an older person with frailty is not always straightforward. Frailty syndromes such as falls, delirium and reduced mobility can mask serious underlying illness. Care and support plans need to be reviewed regularly and in partnership with others, including the person and those important to them, taking account of the changing needs and wishes of the person. Where an older person has been identified as having frailty, it is important to establish systems to share health record information (including the PCP) between primary care, emergency services, secondary care and social services.

Notes

1 www.frailtyfocus.nhs.uk/carers-volunteer.
2 www.scie.org.uk/care-act-2014/assessment-and-eligibility/eligibility/criteria-carers-needs.asp.
3 www.nhs.uk/conditions/social-care-and-support/carers-rights-care-act-2014.
4 http://nuffieldbioethics.org/wp-content/uploads/Dementia-Chapter-6-Dilemmas-in-care.pdf.
5 www.england.nhs.uk/personal-health-budgets.
6 www.nice.org.uk/guidance/ng56/chapter/recommendations.
7 https://ec.europa.eu/research/innovation-union/pdf/active-healthy-ageing/a3_action_plan.pdf.
8 www.caregiver.org/saying-yes-offers-help.
9 www.makingeverycontactcount.co.uk.
10 www.bgs.org.uk/frailty-routine-sit/resources/campaigns/fit-for-frailty/frailty-identify-routine-situation.
11 http://prisma-qc.ca/documents/document/frailelderlypatients.pdf.
12 11 June 2014, www.bgs.org.uk/recognise-frailty-syndrome/resources/campaigns/fit-for-frailty/frailty-frailty-syndromes.
13 www.who.int/about/mission/en.

14 www.england.nhs.uk/ourwork/part-rel/transformation-fund.

15 https://carers.org/what-carer.

16 Clegg A, Young J, Bower P, Cundill B, Farrin A, Foster M, Foy R, Hartley S, Hawkins R, Holmes J, Hulme C, Humphrey S, Lawton R, Pendleton N, West R, Bates C, Nazroo J. Personalised care planning to improve quality of life for older people with frailty. NIHR PGfAR, £2.7 million (October 2017 to February 2023).

References

Ahmed N, Mandel R, Fain MJ. (2007). Frailty: an emerging geriatric syndrome. *Am J Med*. September; 120(9): 748–53.

Andrew MK, Rockwood K. (2010). Social vulnerability predicts cognitive decline in a prospective cohort of older Canadians. *Alzheimers Dement*. 6, 319–25.e1.

Andrew MK, Fisk JD, Rockwood K. (2012). Psychological well-being in relation to frailty: a frailty identity crisis? *Int Psychogeriatr*. August; 24(8): 1347–53. doi:10.1017/S1041610212000269. Epub 2012 March 21.

Anstey KJ, Dixon RA. (2014). Applying a cumulative deficit model of frailty to dementia: progress and future challenges. *Alzheimers Res Ther*. November 26; 6(9): 84. doi:10.1186/s13195-014-0084-z. eCollection 2014.

Antonovsky A. (1987). *Unravelling the mystery of health: how people manage stress and stay well*. San Francisco: Josey-Bass.

Antonovsky A. (1996). The salutogenic model as a theory to guide health promotion. *Health Promotion International*. 11(1): 11–18.

Archibald MM, Ambagtsheer R, Beilby J, Chehade MJ, Gill TK, Visvanathan R, Kitson AL. (2017). Perspectives of frailty and frailty screening: protocol for a collaborative knowledge translation approach and qualitative study of stakeholder understandings and experiences. *BMC Geriatr*. April 17; 17(1): 87. doi:10.1186/s12877-017-0483-7.

Armstrong JJ, Andrew MK, Mitnitski A, Launer LJ, White LR, Rockwood K. (2015). Social vulnerability and survival across levels of frailty in the Honolulu-Asia Aging Study. *Age Ageing*. July; 44(4): 709–12. doi:10.1093/ageing/afv016. Epub 2015 March 10.

Aspinwall LG, MacNamara A. (2005). Taking positive changes seriously. *Cancer*. 104: 2549–56.

Baltes PB. (1997). On the incomplete architecture of human ontogeny. *American Psychologist*. 52: 366–80.

Baum F. (2000). Social capital, economic capital and power: further issues for a public health agenda. *Journal of Epidemiology & Community Health*. 54(6): 409–10.

Bayer R. (2008). Stigma and the ethics of public health: not can we but should we. *Soc Sci Med*. August; 67(3): 463–72. doi:10.1016/j.socscimed.2008.03.017. Epub 2008 May 24.

Bisschop MI, Kriegsman DM, Beekman AT, Deeg DJ. (2004). Chronic diseases and depression: the modifying role of psychosocial resources. *Social Science & Medicine*. 59(4): 721–33. doi:10.1016/j.socscimed.2003.11.038.

Bjorklund R. (1996). Psychiatric labels: still hard to shake. *Psychiatric Services*. 47: 1329–30.

Bonanno GA, Galea S, Bucciarelli A, Ylahov D. (2006). Psychological resilience after disaster: New York city in the aftermath of the September 11th terrorist attack. *Psychological Science*. 17: 181–6.

Bortz WM II. (2002). A conceptual framework of frailty: a review. *J Gerontol A Biol Sci Med Sci*. 57(5): M283–M288.

Bridges J, Flatley M, Meyer J. (2010). Older people's and relatives' experiences in acute care settings: systematic review and synthesis of qualitative studies. *Int J Nurs Stud*. January; 47(1): 89–107. doi:10.1016/j.ijnurstu.2009.09.009. Epub 2009 October 24.

British Geriatrics Society (2014). Fit for frailty. www.bgs.org.uk/fit-for-frailty/resources/campaigns/fit-for-frailty/fff-headlines.

Brouwers C, Merten H, Willems M, Habraken DJ, Bloemers FW, Biesheuvel TH, van Galen LS, Nanayakkara PWB, Wagner C. (2017). Improving care for older patients in the acute setting: a qualitative study with healthcare providers. *Neth J Med*. October; 75(8): 335–43.

Bruyère O, Buckinx F, Beaudart C, Reginster JY, Bauer J, Cederholm T, Cherubini A, Cooper C, Cruz-Jentoft AJ, Landi F, Maggi S, Rizzoli R, Sayer AA, Sieber C, Vellas B, Cesari M; ESCEO and the EUGMS frailty working group. (2017). How clinical practitioners assess frailty in their daily practice: an international survey. *Aging Clin Exp Res*. October; 29(5): 905–12. doi:10.1007/s40520-017-0806-8. Epub 2017 August 2.

Buchner DM, Wagner EH. (1992). Preventing frail health. *Clin. Geriatr. Med.* February; 8(1): 1–17.

Bunt S, Steverink N, Andrew MK, Schans CPV, Hobbelen H. (2017). Cross-cultural adaptation of the Social Vulnerability Index for use in the Dutch Context. *Int J Environ Res Public Health*. November 14; 14(11). pii: E1387. doi:10.3390/ijerph14111387.

Buurman BM, Frenkel WJ, Abu-Hanna A, Parlevliet JL, de Rooij SE. (2016). Acute and chronic diseases as part of multimorbidity in acutely hospitalized older patients. *Eur J Intern Med*. January; 27: 68–75. doi:10.1016/j.ejim.2015.09.021. Epub 2015 October 21.

Cardona OD. (2004). The need for rethinking the concepts of vulnerability and risk from a holistic perspective: A necessary review and criticism for effective risk management. In: Bankoff G, Frerks G, Hilhorst D (eds), *Mapping vulnerability: disasters, development and people*. London, Sterling & VA: Earthscan, Chap. 3. https://doms.csu.edu.au/csu/file/78a6c5d7-fd8b-ff7e-fff3-2ffb78764ebe/1/resources/readings/Reading12_2.pdf.

Carlson JL. 2003. *Complementary therapies and wellness: practice: essentials for holistic health care*. New York: Putnam Hospital Center, Carmel.

Cesari M, Perez-Zepeda MU, Marzetti E. (2017). Frailty and multimorbidity: different ways of thinking about geriatrics. *Journal of the American Medical Directors Association*. 18: 361–4.

Charney DS. (2004). Psychobiological mechanisms of resilience and vulnerability: implications for successful adaptation to extreme stress. *Am J Psychiatry*. February; 161(2): 195–216.

Chen X, Mao G, Leng SX. (2014). Frailty syndrome: an overview. *Clin. Interv. Aging*. http://dx.doi.org/10.2147/cia.s45300.

Chivers S. 2003. *From old woman to older women: contemporary culture and women's narratives*. Columbus, Ohio: Ohio State University Press.

Chochinov HM, McClement S, Hack T, Thompson G, Dufault B, Harlos M. (2015). Eliciting personhood within clinical practice: effects on patients, families, and health care providers. *J Pain Symptom Manage*. June; 49(6): 974–80.e2. doi:10.1016/j.jpainsymman.2014.11.291. Epub 2014 December 17.

Clegg A, Young J, Iliffe S, Rikkert MO, Rockwood K. (2013). Frailty in elderly people, *Lancet*. 381(9868): 752–62.

Conroy SP, Turpin S. (2016). New horizons: urgent care for older people with frailty. *Age Ageing*. September; 45(5): 577–84. doi:10.1093/ageing/afw135. Epub 2016 August 1.

Conti AA, Conti A. (2010). Frailty and resilience from physics to medicine. *Med Hypotheses*. June; 74(6): 1090. doi:10.1016/j.mehy.2010.01.030. Epub 2010 February 18.

Corrigan PW, Bink AB, Schmidt A, Jones N, Rüsch N (2016). What is the impact of self-stigma? Loss of self-respect and the 'why try' effect. *J Ment Health*. 25: 10–15.

Cumming E. (1968). New thoughts on the theory of disengagement. *International Journal of Psychiatry*. 6: 53–67.

DeMartinis M, Franceschi C, Monti D, Ginaldi L. (2006). Inflammation markers predicting frailty and mortality in the elderly. *Exp. Mol. Pathol.* June; 80(3): 219–27. Epub 2006 February 7.

Dent E, Hoogendijk EO. (2014). Psychosocial factors modify the association of frailty with adverse outcomes: a prospective study of hospitalised older people. *BMC Geriatrics.* 14: 108.

Department of Health. (2012). *Long term conditions compendium of information,* 3rd edn. Leeds: Department of Health.

Ebrahimi Z, Wilhelmson K, Eklund K, Moore CD, Jakobsson A. (2013). Health despite frailty: exploring influences on frail older adults' experiences of health. *Geriatr Nurs.* July–August; 34(4): 289–94. doi:10.1016/j.gerinurse.2013.04.008. Epub 2013 May 10.

Feinstein AR. (1970). The pre-therapeutic classification of co-morbidity in chronic disease. *J Chronic Dis.* 23: 455–68.

Fillit H, Butler RN. (2009). The frailty identity crisis. *Journal of the American Geriatrics Society.* 57: 348–52.

Foot J, Hopkins T. (2010). A glass half-full: how an asset approach can improve community health and well-being. (Great Britain Improvement and Development Agency). www.gloucesterpartnership.org.uk/Docs/Glass%20Half%20Full.pdf.

Ford JC, Ford JA. (2017). Multimorbidity: will it stand the test of time? *Age Ageing.* September 26: 1–3. doi:10.1093/ageing/afx159. [Epub ahead of print].

Fortin M, Stewart M, Poitras ME, Almirall J, Maddocks H. (2012). A systematic review of prevalence studies on multimorbidity: toward a more uniform methodology. *Ann Fam Med.* March–April; 10(2): 142–51. doi:10.1370/afm.1337.

Franceschi C, Bonafe M, Valensin S, Olivieri F, De LM, Ottaviani E, De BG. (2000). Inflamm-aging: an evolutionary perspective on immunosenescence. *Ann. N Y Acad. Sci.* 908: 244–54.

Franklin TB, Saab BJ, Mansuy IM. (2012). Neural mechanisms of stress resilience and vulnerability. *Neuron.* September 6; 75(5): 747–61. doi:10.1016/j.neuron.2012.08.016. Review.

Fried LP, Tangen CM, Walston J, Newman AB, Hirsch C, Gottdiener J, Seeman T, Tracy R, Kop WJ, Burke G, McBurnie MA; Cardiovascular Health Study Collaborative Research Group. (2001). Frailty in older adults: evidence for a phenotype. *J Gerontol A Biol Sci Med Sci.* March; 56(3): M146–56.

Friedli L, Parsonage M. (2009). Building an economic case for mental health promotion: Part I. *Journal of Public Mental Health.* 6(3): 14–23.

Frost R, Belk C, Jovicic A, Ricciardi F, Kharicha K, Gardner B, Iliffe S, Goodman C, Manthorpe J, Drennan VM, Walters K. (2017). Health promotion interventions for community-dwelling older people with mild or pre-frailty: a systematic review and meta-analysis. *BMC Geriatr.* July 20; 17(1): 157. doi:10.1186/s12877-017-0547-8.

Fulop T, Larbi A, Witkowski JM, McElhaney J, Loeb M, Mitnitski A, Pawelec G. (2010). Aging, frailty and age-related diseases. *Biogerontology.* October; 11(5): 547–63. doi:10.1007/s10522-010 9287-2. Epub 2010 June 18.

Gale CR, Booth T, Starr JM, Deary IJ. (2016). Intelligence and socioeconomic position in childhood in relation to frailty and cumulative allostatic load in later life: the Lothian Birth Cohort 1936. *J Epidemiol Community Health.* June; 70(6): 576–82. doi:10.1136/jech-2015-205789. Epub 2015 December 23.

Gijzel SMW, van de Leemput IA, Scheffer M, Roppolo M, Olde Rikkert MGM, Melis RJF. (2017). Dynamical resilience indicators in time series of self-rated health correspond to frailty levels in older adults. *J Gerontol A Biol Sci Med Sci.* July 1; 72(7): 991–6. doi:10.1093/gerona/glx065.

Glazer GL, Pressler JL. (1989). Schlotfeldt's health seeking nursing model. In: Fitzpatrick JJ, Whall AL (eds), *Conceptual models of nursing: analysis and application.* Norwalk, CT: Appleton & Lange, pp. 241–53.

Gobbens RJJ, van Assen MALM, Luijkx KG, Wijnen-Sponselee MT, Schols JMGA. (2010). Determinants of frailty. *Journal of the American Medical Directors Association.* 11: 356–64. doi:10.1016/j.jamda.2009.11.008.

Goffman E. (1963). *Stigma: notes on the management of spoiled identity.* New York: Simon and Schuster.

Gompertz B. (1825). On the nature of the function expressive of the law of human mortality and on a new model of determining life contingencies. *Phil Trans R Soc.* 115: 513–85.

Green G. (2009). *The end of stigma? Changes in the social experience of long-term illness.* Abingdon, Oxford: Routledge.

Hardy SE, Concato J, Gill TM. (2002). Stressful life events among community living older persons. *Journal of General Internal Medicine.* 17: 832–8.

Harrison D, Ziglio E, Levin L, Morgan A. (2004). *Assets for health and development: Developing a conceptual framework.* European Office for Investment for Health and Development. Venice: WHO.

Harrison JK, Clegg A, Conroy SP, Young J. (2015). Managing frailty as a long-term condition. *Age Ageing.* September; 44(5): 732–5. doi:10.1093/ageing/afv085. Epub 2015 July 13.

Haslam N. Dehumanization: an integrative review. (2006). *Pers Soc Psychol Rev.* 10(3): 252–64.

Hayne YM. (2003). Experiencing psychiatric diagnosis: client perspectives on being named mentally ill. *J Psychiatr Ment Health Nurs.* December; 10(6): 722–9.

Herek GM, Glunt EK. (1988). An epidemic of stigma: public reactions to AIDS. *American Psychologist.* 43: 886–91.

Hindhede AL, Aagaard-Hansen J. (2017). Using social network analysis as a method to assess and strengthen participation in health promotion programs in vulnerable areas. *Health Promot Pract.* March; 18(2): 175–83. doi:10.1177/1524839916686029. Epub 2017 January 24.

Holt-Lunstad J, Smith TB, Layton JB. (2010). Social relationships and mortality risk: a meta-analytic review. *Plos Medicine.* July; 7(7). doi:10.1371/journal.pmed.1000316.

Hoogendijk EO, Theou O, Rockwood K, Onwuteaka-Philipsen BD, Deeg DJH, Huisman M. (2017). Development and validation of a frailty index in the Longitudinal Aging Study Amsterdam. *Aging Clin Exp Res.* October; 29(5): 927–33. doi:10.1007/s40520-016-0689-0. Epub 2016 November 28.

Hoogendijk EO, van Hout HP, van der Horst HE, Frijters DH, Dent E, Deeg DJ, Huisman M. (2014). Do psychosocial resources modify the effects of frailty on functional decline and mortality? *Journal of Psychosomatic Research.* 77(6): 547–51. doi:10.1016/j.jpsychores.2014.09.017.

Hornby-Turner YC, Peel NM, Hubbard RE. (2017). Health assets in older age: a systematic review. *BMJ Open.* May 17; 7(5): e013226. doi:10.1136/bmjopen-2016-013226.

Howlett SE, Rockwood K. (2013). New horizons in frailty: ageing and the deficit-scaling problem. *Age Ageing.* July; 42(4): 416–23. doi:10.1093/ageing/aft059. Epub 2013 June 5.

Hubbard R, Ng K; Australian and New Zealand Society for Geriatric Medicine. (2015). Australian and New Zealand Society for Geriatric Medicine: position statement – frailty in older people. *Australas J Ageing.* Mar; 34(1): 68–73. doi:10.1111/ajag.12195.

Hubbard RE, Goodwin VA, Llewellyn DJ, Warmoth K, Lang IA. (2014). Frailty, financial resources and subjective well-being in later life. *Archives of Gerontology and Geriatrics.* 58(3): 364–9. doi: 10.1016/j.archger.2013.12.008.

Huber M, Knottnerus JA, Green L, van der Horst H, Jadad AR, Kromhout D, Leonard B, Lorig K, Loureiro MI, van der Meer JW, Schnabel P, Smith R, van Weel C, Smid H. (2011). How should we define health? *BMJ*. July 26; 343: d4163. doi:10.1136/bmj. d4163.

Huffman DM, Justice JN, Stout MB, Kirkland JL, Barzilai N, Austad SN. (2016). Evaluating health span in preclinical models of aging and disease: guidelines, challenges, and opportunities for geroscience. *J Gerontol A Biol Sci Med Sci*. November; 71(11): 1395–406. Epub 2016 August 16.

Islam MK, Merlo J, Kawachi I, Lindström M, Gerdtham U-G. (2006). Social capital and health: does egalitarianism matter? A literature review. *International Journal for Equity in Health*. 5(3). doi:10.1186/1475-9276-5-3.

Kawachi I. (2010). The relationship between health assets, social capital and cohesive communities. In: Morgan A, Davies M, Ziglio E (eds), *Health assets in a global context*. New York: Springer, pp. 167–79.

Kessing D, Pelle AJ, Kupper N, Szabo BM, Denollet J. (2014). Positive affect, anhedonia, and compliance with self-care in patients with chronic heart failure. *Journal of Psychosomatic Research*. 77(4): 296–301. doi:10.1016/j.jpsychores.2014.08.007.

Keusch GT, Wilentz J, Kleinman A. (2006). Stigma and global health: developing a research agenda. *Lancet*. February 11; 367(9509): 525–7.

Kim D, Subramanian SV, Kawachi I. (2007). Social capital and physical health: a systematic review of the literature. In: Kawachi I, Subramanian SV, Kim D (eds), *Social capital and health*. New York: Springer, pp. 139–90.

Kirby SE, Coleman PG, Daley D. (2004). Spirituality and well-being in frail and nonfrail older adults. *The Journals of Gerontology Series B: Psychological Sciences and Social Sciences*. 59(3): 123–9. doi: 10.1093/geronb/59.3.P123.

Kogan AC, Wilber K, Mosqueda L. (2016). Person-centered care for older adults with chronic conditions and functional impairment: a systematic literature review. *J Am Geriatr Soc*. January; 64(1): e1–7. doi:10.1111/jgs.13873. Epub 2015 December 2.

Kretzmann JP, McKnight JL. (1993). *Building communities from the inside out: a path toward finding and mobilizing a community's assets*. Evanston, IL: Institute for Policy Research.

Lang IA, Hubbard RE, Andrew MK, Llewellyn DJ, Melzer D, Rockwood K. (2009). Neighborhood deprivation, individual socioeconomic status, and frailty in older adults. *J Am Geriatr Soc*. October; 57(10): 1776–80. doi:10.1111/j.1532-5415.2009.02480.x. Epub 2009 September 15.

Lang PO, Michel JP, Zekry D. (2009). Frailty syndrome: a transitional state in a dynamic process. *Gerontology*. 55(5): 539–49. doi:10.1159/000211949. Epub 2009 April 4.

Lazarus RS, Folkman S. (1984). *Stress, appraisal, and coping*. New York: Springer.

Le Lain R, Ignaszewski C, Klingmann I, Cesario A, de Boer WI; SPRINTT Consortium. (2017). SPRINTT and the involvement of stakeholders: strategy and structure. *Aging Clin Exp Res*. February; 29(1): 65–7. doi:10.1007/s40520-016-0706-3. Epub 2017 January 31.

Levy R. (2009). Stereotype embodiment: a psychosocial approach to aging. *Current Directions in Psychological Science*. 18(6): 332–6.

Lindstrom B, Eriksson M. (2005). Salutogenesis. *Journal of Epidemiology and Community Health*. 59(6): 440–2.

Link BG, Phelan JC. (2001). Conceptualizing stigma. *Annual Review of Sociology*. 27: 363–85.

Luthar SS, Cicchetti D, Becker B. (2000). The construct of resilience: a critical evaluation and guidelines for future work. *Child Dev*. May–June; 71(3): 543–62.

Magis K. (2010). Community resilience: an indicator of social sustainability. *Society and Natural Resources*. 23(5): 401–16.

Manton KG, Woodbury MA, Stallard E. (1995). Sex differences in human mortality and aging at late ages: the effect of mortality selection and state dynamics. *The Gerontologist.* 35: 597–608.

Marmot M. (2010). *Fair society, healthy lives: strategic review of health inequalities in England post 2010* (The Marmot Review). London: Institute of Health Equity.

Marmot M, Friel S, Bell R, Houweling TAJ, Taylor S. (2008). Closing the gap in a generation: health equity through action on the social determinants of health. *Lancet.* 372: 1661–9.

McCusker J, Verdon J, Vadeboncoeur A, Lévesque JF, Sinha SK, Kim KY, Belzile E. (2012). The elder-friendly emergency department assessment tool: development of a quality assessment tool for emergency department-based geriatric care. *J Am Geriatr Soc.* August; 60(8): 1534–9. doi:10.1111/j.1532-5415.2012.04058.x. Epub 2012 August 2.

Meeks S, Van Haitsma K, Mast BT, Arnold S, Streim JE, Sephton S, Rovine M. (2016). Psychological and social resources relate to biomarkers of allostasis in newly admitted nursing home residents. *Aging and Mental Health.* 20(1): 88–99.

Ménard C, Pfau ML, Hodes GE, Russo SJ. (2017). Immune and neuroendocrine mechanisms of stress vulnerability and resilience. *Neuropsychopharmacology.* January; 42(1): 62–80. doi:10.1038/npp. 2016.90. Epub 2016 June 13.

Mitnitski AB, Mogilner AJ, Rockwood K. (2001). Accumulation of deficits as a proxy measure of aging. *Scientific World Journal.* 1: 323–36.

Mitnitski AB, Rutenberg AD, Farrell S, Rockwood K. (2017). Aging, frailty and complex networks. *Biogerontology.* March 2. doi:10.1007/s10522-017-9684-x. [Epub ahead of print] Review.

Mitnitski A, Song X, Rockwood K. (2013). Assessing biological aging: the origin of deficit accumulation. *Biogerontology.* December; 14(6): 709–17. doi:10.1007/s10522-013-9446-3. Epub 2013 July 17.

Moore T, Huerena J. (2005). Can you really be healthy as a person with a disability? In: Nehring WM (ed.), *Health promotion for persons with intellectual and developmental disabilities: the state of scientific evidence.* Washington, DC: American Association on Mental Retardation, pp. 343–6.

Morgan A, Hernán M. (2013). Promoting health and wellbeing through the asset model. [Article in English, Spanish]. *Rev Esp Sanid Penit.* February; 15(3): 78–86. doi:10.4321/S1575-06202013000300001.

Morgan A, Ziglio E. (2007). Revitalising the evidence base for public health: an assets model. *Promot Educ.* 14(Suppl. 2): 17–22.

Murphy C, Gardoni P. (2006). The role of society in engineering risk analysis: a capabilities-based approach. *Risk Anal.* August; 26(4): 1073–83.

NIHR Dissemination Centre. (2017). Themed review. Comprehensive care: older people living with frailty in hospitals. www.dc.nihr.ac.uk/themed-reviews/Comprehensive-Care-final.pdf.

Norton B, McLeroy K, Burdine J. (2002). Community capacity: concept, theory and methods. In: DiClemente R, Crosby R, Kegler M (eds), *Emerging theories in health promotion practice and research.* San Francisco: Jossey-Bass, pp. 194–227.

Nunes BP, Flores TR, Mielke GI, Thumé E, Facchini LA. (2016). Multimorbidity and mortality in older adults: a systematic review and meta-analysis. *Arch Gerontol Geriatr.* November–December; 67: 130–8. doi:10.1016/j.archger.2016.07.008. Epub 2016 August 2.

Orlando Frailty Conference Group. (2013). Raising awareness on the urgent need to implement frailty into clinical practice. *J Frailty Aging.* September; 2(3): 121–4.

Ottenvall Hammar I, Dahlin-Ivanoff S, Wilhelmson K, Eklund K. (2014). Shifting between self-governing and being governed: a qualitative study of older persons' self-determination. *BMC Geriatr.* November 28; 14: 126. doi:10.1186/1471-2318-14-126.

Penrod J, Baney B, Loeb SJ, McGhan G, Shipley PZ. (2012). The influence of the culture of care on informal caregivers' experiences. *ANS Adv Nurs Sci.* January–March; 35(1): 64–76. doi:10.1097/ANS.0b013e318244555a.

Pescosolido BA, Martin JK, Lang A, Olafsdottir S. (2008). Rethinking theoretical approaches to stigma: a Framework Integrating Normative Influences on Stigma (FINIS). *Soc Sci Med.* August; 67(3): 431–40. doi:10.1016/j.socscimed.2008.03.018. Epub 2008 April 22.

Podsiadlo D, Richardson S. (1991) The timed 'Up & Go': a test of basic functional mobility for frail elderly persons. *J Am Geriatr Soc.* February; 39(2): 142–8.

Pons-Vigués M, Berenguera A, Coma-Auli N, Pombo-Ramos H, March S, Asensio-Martínez A, Moreno-Peral P, Mora-Simón S, Martínez-Andrés M, Pujol-Ribera E. (2017). Health-care users, key community informants and primary health care workers' views on health, health promotion, health assets and deficits: qualitative study in seven Spanish regions. *Int J Equity Health.* June 13; 16(1): 99. doi:10.1186/s12939-017-0590-2.

Popay J, Attree P, Hornby D, Milton B, Whitehead M, French B, Kowarzik U, Simpson N, Povall S. (2007). *Community engagement in initiatives addressing the wider social determinants of health: a rapid review of evidence on impact, experience and process.* Lancaster: Universities of Lancaster, Liverpool and Central Lancashire.

Puchalski CM, Jafari N. (2015). Acknowledging the person in the clinical encounter: whole person care for patients and clinicians alike. Commentary on Chochinov *et al. J Pain Symptom Manage.* June; 49(6): 973. doi:10.1016/j.jpainsymman.2015.04.008. Epub 2015 May 1.

Radner H, Yoshida K, Smolen JS, Solomon DH. (2014). Multimorbidity and rheumatic conditions enhancing the concept of comorbidity. *Nat Rev Rheumatol.* 10: 252–6.

Raîche M, Hébert R, Dubois MF. (2007). PRISMA-7: a case-finding tool to identify older adults with moderate to severe disabilities. *Arch Gerontol Geriatr.* 2008 Jul–Aug; 47(1): 9–18. Epub 2007 August 27.

Reingold AL, Krishnan S. (2001, September). The study of potentially stigmatizing conditions: an epidemiologic perspective. Paper presented at the National Institutes of Health International Stigma Conference, Bethesda, MD.

Ritt M, Gaßmann KG, Sieber CC. (2016). Significance of frailty for predicting adverse clinical outcomes in different patient groups with specific medical conditions. *Z Gerontol Geriatr.* October; 49(7): 567–72. Epub 2016 September 14.

Rockwood K. (2005). What would make a definition of frailty successful? *Age and Ageing.* 34(5): 432–4.

Rockwood K, Hubbard R. (2004). Frailty and the geriatrician. *Age and Ageing.* September; 33(5): 429–30. No abstract available.

Rockwood K, Mitnitski A. (2006). Limits to deficit accumulation in elderly people. *Mech Ageing Dev.* May; 127(5): 494–6. Epub 2006 February 20.

Rockwood K, Mitnitski A. (2007). Frailty in relation to the accumulation of deficits. *J Gerontol A Biol Sci Med Sci.* 62: 722–7.

Rockwood K, Mitnitski A. (2011). Frailty defined by deficit accumulation and geriatric medicine defined by frailty. *Clin Geriatr Med.* February; 27(1): 17–26. doi:10.1016/j.cger.2010.08.008.

Rockwood K, Fox RA, Stolee P, Robertson D, Beattie BL. (1994). Frailty in elderly people: an evolving concept. *Canadian Medical Association Journal.* 150(4): 489–95.

Rockwood K, Mitnitski A, Song X, Steen B, Skoog I. (2006). Long-term risks of death and institutionalization of elderly people in relation to deficit accumulation at age 70. *J Am Geriatr Soc.* June; 54(6): 975–9.

Rockwood K, Mogilner A, Mitnitski A (2004). Changes with age in the distribution of a frailty index. *Mech Ageing Dev.* 125: 517–19.

Rodríguez-Mañas L, Féart C, Mann G, Viña J, Chatterji S, Chodzko-Zajko W, Gonzalez-Colaço Harmand M, Bergman H, Carcaillon L, Nicholson C, Scuteri A, Sinclair A, Pelaez M, Van der Cammen T, Beland F, Bickenbach J, Delamarche P, Ferrucci L, Fried LP, Gutiérrez-Robledo LM, Rockwood K, Rodríguez Artalejo F, Serviddio G, Vega E; FOD-CC group (Appendix 1). (2013). Searching for an operational definition of frailty: a Delphi method based consensus statement: the frailty operative definition-consensus conference project. *J Gerontol A Biol Sci Med Sci.* January; 68(1): 62–7. doi:10.1093/gerona/gls119. Epub 2012 April 16.

Rogers W, Mackenzie C, Dodds S. (2012). Why bioethics needs a concept of vulnerability. *International Journal of Feminist Approaches to Bioethics.* 5(2): 11–38.

Rotegård AK, Moore SM, Fagermoen MS, Ruland CM. (2010). Health assets: a concept analysis. *Int J Nurs Stud.* April; 47(4): 513–25. doi:10.1016/j.ijnurstu.2009.09.005. Epub 2009 October 12.

Routasalo PE, Tilvis RS, Kautiainen H, Pitkala KH. (2009). Effects of psychosocial group rehabilitation on social functioning, loneliness and well-being of lonely, older people: randomized controlled trial. *Journal of Advanced Nursing.* 65(2): 297–305.

Rowe J, Kahn R. (1998). *Successful aging.* New York: Random House.

Rowe JW, Kahn RL. (2015). Successful aging 2.0: conceptual expansions for the 21st century. *Journals of Gerontology, Series B: Psychological Sciences and Social Sciences.* 70(4): 593–6. doi:10.1093/geronb/gbv025.

Sabia S, Singh-Manoux A, Hagger-Johnson G, Cambois E, Brunner EJ, Kivimaki M. (2012). Influence of individual and combined healthy behaviours on successful aging. *Canadian Medical Association Journal.* 184(18): 1985–92.

Sales AE. (2009). Comorbidities, frailty, and 'pay-off time'. *Med Care.* June; 47(6): 607–9. doi:10.1097/MLR.0b013e3181a5c629.

Scambler G. (2009). Health-related stigma. *Sociol Health Illn.* April; 31(3): 441–55. doi:10.1111/j.1467-9566.2009.01161.x.

Schoenborn NL, Van Pilsum Rasmussen SE, Xue QL, Walston JD, McAdams-Demarco MA, Segev DL, Boyd CM. (2018). Older adults' perceptions and informational needs regarding frailty. *BMC Geriatr.* February 13; 18(1): 46. doi:10.1186/s12877-018-0741-3.

Schulz R, Heckhausen J. (1996). A life span model of successful aging. *American Psychologist.* 51(7): 702–14.

Searle SD, Mitnitski A, Gahbauer EA, Gill TM, Rockwood K (2008). A standard procedure for creating a frailty index. *BMC Geriatr.* 8: 24.

Shankar A, Hamer M, McMunn A, Steptoe A. (2013). Social isolation and loneliness: relationships with cognitive function during 4 years of follow-up in the English Longitudinal Study of Ageing. *Psychosom Med.* February; 75(2): 161–70. doi:10.1097/PSY.0b013e31827f09cd. Epub 2013 January 29.

Shears M, McGolrick D, Waters B, Jakab M, Boyd JG, Muscedere J. (2017). Frailty measurement and outcomes in interventional studies: protocol for a systematic review of randomised control trials. *BMJ Open.* December 26; 7(12): e018872. doi:10.1136/bmjopen-2017-018872.

Sherman CW, Webster NJ, Antonucci TC. (2013). Dementia caregiving in the context of late-life remarriage: support networks, relationship quality, and well-being. *Journal of Marriage and Family.* 75: 1149–63.

Sieber CC. (2017). Frailty: from concept to clinical practice. *Exp Gerontol.* January; 87(Pt B): 160–7. doi:10.1016/j.exger.2016.05.004. Epub 2016 May 17.

Silva CF, Howe PD. (2012). Difference, adapted physical activity and human development: potential contribution of capabilities approach. *Adapt Phys Activ Q.* January; 29(1): 25–43.

Song X, Mitnitski A, Rockwood K. (2010). Prevalence and 10-year outcomes of frailty in older adults in relation to deficit accumulation. *J Am Geriatr Soc.* April; 58(4): 681–7. doi:10.1111/j.1532-5415.2010.02764.x. Epub 2010 March 22.

Song X, Mitnitski A, Rockwood K. (2014). Age-related deficit accumulation and the risk of late-life dementia. *Alzheimers Res Ther.* September 18; 6(5–8): 54. doi:10.1186/s13195-014-0054-5. eCollection 2014.

Soysal P, Isik AT, Carvalho AF, Fernandes BS, Solmi M, Schofield P, Veronese N, Stubbs B. (2017). Oxidative stress and frailty: a systematic review and synthesis of the best evidence. *Maturitas.* May; 99: 66–72. doi:10.1016/j.maturitas.2017.01.006. Epub 2017 January 16.

Steptoe A, Deaton A, Stone AA. (2015). Subjective wellbeing, health, and ageing. *Lancet.* 385(9968): 640–8. doi:10.1016/s0140-6736(13)61489-0.

Steunenberg B, Beekman AT, Deeg DJ, Bremmer MA, Kerkhof AJ. (2007). Mastery and neuroticism predict recovery of depression in later life. *American Journal of Geriatric Psychiatry.* 15(3): 234–42. doi:10.1097/01.JGP.0000236595.98623.62.

Steverink N, Westerhof GJ, Bode C, Dittmann-Kohli F. (2001). The personal experience of aging, individual resources, and subjective well-being. *The Journals of Gerontology Series B: Psychological Sciences and Social Sciences.* 56: 364–73.

Taylor SE, Stanton AL. (2007). Coping resources, coping processes, and mental health. *Annual Review of Clinics Psychological.* 3: 377–401.

Tinetti ME, Fried T. (2004). The end of the disease era. *Am J Med.* February 1; 116(3): 179–85.

Varadhan R, Walston JD, Bandeen-Roche K. (2018). Can a link be found between physical resilience and frailty in older adults by studying dynamical systems? *J Am Geriatr Soc.* May 4. doi:10.1111/jgs.15409. [Epub ahead of print].

Velanovich V, Antoine H, Swartz A, Peters D, Rubinfeld I. (2013). Accumulating deficits model of frailty and postoperative mortality and morbidity: its application to a national database. *J Surg Res.* July; 183(1): 104–10. doi:10.1016/j.jss.2013.01.021. Epub 2013 February 1.

Vetrano DL, Foebel AD, Marengoni A, Brandi V, Collamati A, Heckman GA, Hirdes J, Bernabei R, Onder G. (2016). Chronic diseases and geriatric syndromes: the different weight of comorbidity. *Eur J Intern Med.* January; 27: 62–7. doi:10.1016/j.ejim.2015.10.025. Epub 2015 November 28.

Wallace LM, Theou O, Pena F, Rockwood K, Andrew MK. (2015). Social vulnerability as a predictor of mortality and disability: cross-country differences in the Survey of Health, Aging, and Retirement in Europe (SHARE). *Aging Clin Exp Res.* June; 27(3): 365–72. doi:10.1007/s40520-014 0271-6. Epub 2014 September 12.

Warmoth K, Lang I, Phoenix C, Abraham C, Andrew MK, Hubbard RE, Tarrant M. (2016). 'Thinking you're old and frail': a qualitative study of frailty in older adults. *Ageing Soc.* 36(7): 1483–500.

Whiting L, Kendall S, Wills W. (2012). An asset-based approach: an alternative health promotion strategy? *Community Practitioner.* 85(1): 25–8.

Woo J, Goggins W, Sham A, Ho SC. (2005). Social determinants of frailty. *Gerontology.* 51: 402–8.

Woo J, Leung J, Morley JE. (2012). Comparison of frailty indicators based on clinical phenotype and the multiple deficit approach in predicting mortality and physical limitation. *J Am Geriatr Soc.* August; 60(8): 1478–86. doi:10.1111/j.1532 5415.2012.04074.x. Epub 2012 August 2.

Woo J, Leung J, Zhang T. (2016). Successful aging and frailty: opposite sides of the same coin? *J Am Med Dir Assoc.* September 1; 17(9): 797–801. doi:10.1016/j.jamda.2016.04.015. Epub 2016 May 25.

World Health Organization. (1986). *Ottawa charter for health promotion.* Ottawa, Ontario.

World Health Organization. (2012). *Dementia: a public health priority.* Geneva.

Wyrko Z. (2015). Frailty at the front door. *Clin Med* (Lond). August; 15(4): 377–81. doi:10.7861/clinmedicine.15-4-377.

You JJ, Fowler RA, Heyland DK; Canadian Researchers at the End of Life Network (CARENET). (2014). Just ask: discussing goals of care with patients in hospital with serious illness. *CMAJ.* 186: 425–32.

Zozulya AA, Gabaeva MV, Sokolov OY, Surkina ID, Kost NV. (2008). Personality, coping style, and constitutional neuroimmunology. *J. Immunotoxicol.* 5: 221–5.

2

LIVING WELL WITH FRAILTY

From identity to care

Aim

In this chapter, I'd like to look at why quality of life in frailty is so important, and how it can be affected in a selection of medical conditions. I will consider why we should want to identify people who are 'frail' or 'pre-frail' at all, including the pivotal importance of the comprehensive geriatric assessment.

Quality of life in frailty

'If you value it, measure it.' That is one of the best reasons to want to identify and measure quality of life in people who are frail. Maintaining a strong sense of psychological wellbeing in the face of the changes and losses of later life is generally considered a crucial part of '**healthy ageing**' (Baltes and Baltes, 1990). Medicine has a strong influence on how frailty is conceptualised nowadays, meaning that frailty is usually predominantly defined in terms of physical function. However, an increasing number of researchers is currently convinced of the multidimensional nature of frailty (e.g. Gobbens *et al.*, 2017). More generally, as discussed in Chapter 1, it has been proposed that the onset of frailty is associated with an identity crisis, the so-called frailty identity crisis, a psychological syndrome that may accompany the transition from robustness to the 'next to last' stage of life. The psychological challenges stemming from the development of frailty such as regrets, sadness and depression can complicate physical frailty itself and have received little attention in literature so far; therefore, the need for studies on the independent correlates and outcomes of the frailty identity crisis, including quality of life (QOL), has been recently highlighted (Bilotta *et al.*, 2010).

Supporting individual decisions and choices, and supporting self-care, can make a significant contribution to improving quality of life for people living with frailty.

Although most people reckon that they know what quality of life entails (Gilhooly *et al.*, 2005), it can be difficult to define the concept as both objective and subjective aspects influence QOL (Gabriel and Bowling, 2004; Gilhooly *et al.*, 2005). QOL assessment has become increasingly common to supplement the objective measurements of health in clinical research, and is important in assessing the effectiveness of interventions or arriving at treatment decisions (Guyatt *et al.*, 1993). QOL is a generic concept reflecting concern with the modification and enhancement of life attributes, e.g. the physical, moral and social environment; the overall condition of a human life (Gregersen *et al.*, 2015).

In research, QOL is applied both as an objective condition of life which is assumed to have a positive impact upon wellbeing, and as a subjective concept of experienced wellbeing and life satisfaction (Zachariae and Bech, 2008). Currently, studies aimed at enhancing the QOL of older long-term care residents are limited and often directed to physical and psychological interventions. The lack of a systematic effect on QOL is possibly related to the fact that these interventions were often not multidimensional, whereas QOL is a multidimensional concept (Van Malderen *et al.*, 2013).

Measuring quality of life in frailty

Measures of quality of life vary. Having an international quality of life assessment such as the WHOQOL (World Health Organization Quality of Life assessment) makes it possible to carry out quality of life research collaboratively in different cultural settings, and to compare directly results obtained in these different settings (WHO, 1985). The World Health Organization has developed two generic instruments for assessing quality of life, the WHOQOL-100 and its short form the WHOQOL-BREF. However, it became obvious that both instruments were insufficient for the specific requirements of assessing quality of life in old age (Gobbens and Van Assen, 2016). The Older People's QOL Questionnaire (OPQOL) is of potential value in the outcome assessment of health and social interventions, which can have a multidimensional impact on people's lives (Bowling and Stenner, 2011). It is important that measures are appropriate for older adults, as health services become increasingly focused on their needs and resource allocation (Sexton *et al.*, 2017).

Frailty and quality of life – specific examples

Older adults with minor fractures who are frail appear to have lower physical and mental health related quality of life (HRQOL) scores at three and six months after emergency department (ED) discharge than their fittest counterparts (Provencher *et al.*, 2016).

Frailty may lead to a worsening of the patient's QOL, possibly due to a reduction in functional capacity, which increases physical fatigue. Both of these issues reduce the patient's mobility, thus lowering social interaction and generating dependency, which can be aggravated in people with clinical complications such as those related to CKD (chronic kidney disease) (Mansur et al., 2104). Frail survivors of critical illness may experience a markedly worse psychosocial and physical recovery along with a unique spectrum of survivorship problems compared with those who are not frail (Gill et al., 2010).

Frail 'survivors of critical illness' experience greater impairment in health-related quality of life, functional dependence and disability compared with those not frail. The systematic assessment of frailty may assist in better informing patients and families on the complexities of survivorship and recovery (Bagshaw et al., 2015). A recent study, furthermore, demonstrated that frailty is a significant predictor of quality of life in liver transplant candidates. Patients defined as frail, receiving a frailty score of three or more, had significantly worse quality of life scores than the non-frail group (Derck et al., 2015). The presence of frailty has a negative impact on early QOL in patients with acute coronary syndromes (ACS) (Lisiak et al., 2016). The study suggests that in elderly patients with ACS, there is a need to identify frailty in order to implement additional therapeutic and nursing strategies in ACS.

The impact of sarcopenia on quality of life is currently assessed by generic tools. However, these tools may not detect subtle effects of this specific condition on quality of life. the aim of this study was to develop a sarcopenia-specific quality of life questionnaire (SarQOL, Sarcopenia Quality of Life) designed for community-dwelling elderly subjects aged 65 years and older (Beaudart et al., 2015). The first version of the SarQOL has been developed and has been shown to be comprehensible by the target population. Investigations are now required to test the psychometric properties (internal consistency, test–retest reliability, divergent and convergent validity, discriminant validity, floor and ceiling effects) of this questionnaire.

Frailty in some medical conditions

Metabolic syndrome and diabetes

The metabolic syndrome (MetS) results from a combination of risk factors for type 2 diabetes and cardiovascular events. A large body of evidence relates MetS with the risk of premature death (Scuteri et al., 2005; Wang et al., 2007). Older individuals with MetS and diseases such as type 2 diabetes, cardiovascular disease or obesity are more often frail (Blaum et al., 2005; Hubbard et al., 2010; Viscogliosi, 2016). Furthermore, MetS has recently been linked to 'incident frailty' (Viscogliosi, 2016). Diabetes mellitus is associated with higher risk of frailty; this association is partly explained by unhealthy behaviours and obesity and, to a greater extent, by poor glucose control and altered serum lipid profile among diabetic individuals. Conversely, diabetes nutritional therapy reduces the risk of frailty (García-Esquinas et al., 2015). A recent study in very old people (90+ years) showed that while a higher FI score was associated with a greater risk of mortality, metabolic syndrome status was not (Hao et al., 2016).

It seems that, from a recent retrospective cohort study using primary care electronic medical records (the United Kingdom Health Improvement Network Database), glycaemic and systemic blood pressure control are similar for otherwise fit adults with type 2 diabetes mellitus (T2DM) as for patients who are frail (McAlister *et al.*, 2018). Rather surprisingly, however, the literature considering frailty as a risk factor for T2DM is limited. A number of cross-sectional studies have suggested that frail people have a higher prevalence of T2DM, but it is not possible to disentangle the directionality of these associations, particularly given that some studies have demonstrated that T2DM is a risk factor for frailty (Veronese *et al.*, 2016).

Hypoglycaemia causes recurrent hospital admissions because of syncope or fracture and eventually leads to frailty. Hypoglycaemia also leads to cognitive dysfunction, and subsequently physical frailty. Frailty, in turn, is associated with under-nutrition, leading to hypoglycaemia. Therefore, hypoglycaemia and frailty work in a vicious cycle. Hypoglycaemic symptoms tend to be less specific with increasing age (Won and Kim, 2016). In a recent study of elderly patients with diabetes mellitus, low HbA1c was identified to be a significant and independent risk factor for frailty, as assessed using a broad-sense frailty scale, the Clinical Frailty Scale, suggesting that reverse metabolism due to malnutrition in elderly T2DM patients might be involved. Therefore, it is suggested that an intervention that includes proper nutrition and exercise training may be essential for the prevention of frailty (Yanase *et al.*, 2017).

Renal failure

Although chronic renal disease itself is a predictor of adverse health outcomes, coexistence of chronic renal disease and frailty has been shown to further increase risks of falls, fractures, hospitalisation and mortality (Kojima, 2017). Prevalence of frailty among young and elderly end-stage renal disease (ESRD) patients is high; being female and having more comorbidity was associated with frailty. Use of a broader definition of frailty, like the FI, gives a higher estimation of prevalence among ESRD patients compared with a physical frailty assessment.

The relationship between chronic renal disease and frailty is not completely understood yet. Studies have shown that inflammation is associated with frailty in many chronic diseases and this suggests a 'shared pathophysiology' of frailty (Jeffery *et al.*, 2013). In particular, the pro-inflammatory cytokines interleukin-6 and tumour necrosis factor alpha may have a role in age-related muscle atrophy and sarcopenia, which are key features of frailty (Hubbard and Woodhouse, 2010). Shlipak and colleagues (Shlipak *et al.*, 2003) demonstrated that there are raised levels of pro-inflammatory cytokines in patients with chronic renal disease. However, further research is needed to investigate the causal relationship between inflammation and frailty specifically in patients with chronic renal disease. A previous systematic review (studies published up to 2012) had explored frailty in pre-dialysis patients and showed an association between frailty and chronic renal disease (Walker *et al.*, 2013).

Heart failure

At this time, it is not possible to clinically differentiate primary frailty from frailty secondary to chronic disease. With respect to the ageing heart failure (HF) population, there is an urgent need to address the potential for this distinction (Goldwater and Pinney, 2015).

It has been documented there is a bidirectional relationship between frailty and cardiovascular disease, with frailty being a powerful predictor of mortality in cardiac patients (Montero-Odasso *et al.*, 2005). The impact of concurrent frailty and CHF (chronic heart failure) is evident, given that the prevalence of CHF increases six- to seven-fold with increasing frailty severity (Fried *et al.*, 2001; Woods *et al.*, 2005). The elucidation of common pathological processes spanning immunological, metabolic and autonomic systems indicates a multifaceted and complex association between the two syndromes. The high prevalence of frailty in heart failure is well documented, and as such it has been identified as an emergent area of research priority (McDonagh *et al.*, 2017). The reason for this is complex and multifaceted. A number of studies have demonstrated high prevalence rates of frailty in HF and worse associated clinical outcomes among frail adults with HF (Cacciatore *et al.*, 2005; Jha *et al.*, 2016; McNallan *et al.*, 2013; Boxer *et al.*, 2010; Dominguez-Rodriguez *et al.*, 2015).

Commonalities in the pathogenesis of frailty and HF continue to be of interest (see Figure 2.1).

It is sometimes argued that frailty needs to move from a being an 'interesting research variable' to an important clinical instrument utilised as part of the management plan for individuals with HF. At that point, instead of merely predicting worse outcomes, frailty assessment can help prevent them (McDonagh *et al.*, 2018).

HIV/AIDS

As patients living with HIV grow older, some accumulate multiple health problems earlier than the noninfected patients, in particular frailty phenotypes. Patients with frailty phenotype are at higher risk of adverse outcomes (worsening mobility, disability, hospitalisation, and death within three years). Multivariate logistic regression analyses showed that only pain was significantly different between frail and pre-frail phenotype versus non-frail phenotype (Petit *et al.*, 2018). Since HIV patients have seen 'accelerated ageing', it is likely that many people ageing with treated HIV infection may have their physical function affected (Brañas *et al.*, 2017). A higher frailty phenotype prevalence in HIV-infected compared with non-HIV-infected populations has been observed (Desquilbet *et al.*, 2007; Terzian *et al.*, 2009; Pathai *et al.*, 2013).

Among middle-aged and older HIV-infected individuals, including those with well-suppressed infection, frailty and impairments in physical function are common (Gustafson *et al.*, 2016; Levett *et al.*, 2016; Erlandson *et al.*, 2014). Inflammation and immune activation, likely important in the pathophysiology of frailty in the general population (Hubbard *et al.*, 2009; Walston *et al.*, 2002), may be mediating the association between HIV infection and frailty (Margolick *et al.*, 2013; Erlandson *et*

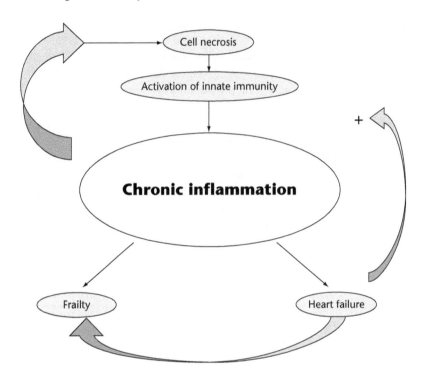

FIGURE 2.1 Frailty and heart failure

Source: redrawn from Figure 1, p. 3 of Bellumkonda L, Tyrrell D, Hummel SL, Goldstein DR. (2017). Pathophysiology of heart failure and frailty: a common inflammatory origin? *Aging Cell*. June; 16(3): 444–50. doi:10.1111/acel.12581. Epub 2017 March 7.

Note
Possible inflammatory pathophysiological link between frailty and HF processes that occur with ageing (e.g. cellular senescence, increased oxidative stress, reduced autophagy or mitophagy, increased DNA damage, or mitochondrial dysfunction) accompany both frailty and HF. These processes may ultimately disrupt cellular homeostasis and lead to cell death.

al., 2013; Erlandson *et al.*, 2014). Both HIV infection by itself, as well as exposure to antiretroviral therapy, may contribute to body composition changes, and thereby to the development of frailty in the context of HIV (Stanley and Grinspoon, 2012). Loss of bone mineral density is observed in the elderly and accelerated by HIV infection and antiretroviral treatment (Brown and Qaqish, 2009). Although a low $CD4^+$ cell count has been observed to be a strong risk factor for frailty among both HIV-infected women and HIV-infected men (in the Multicenter AIDS Cohort Study (MACS)) (Terzian *et al.*, 2009; Desquilbet *et al.*, 2009), subsequent studies in the era of potent combination antiretroviral therapy (cART), have continued to demonstrate a higher prevalence of frailty among HIV-infected compared to non-HIV-infected populations, though lower than in the pre-cART era (Gustafson *et al.*, 2016).

A possible overview of HIV and frailty is shown in Figure 2.2.

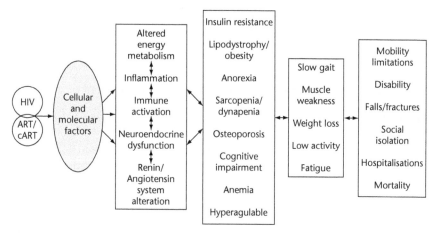

FIGURE 2.2   Potential integrative context around which to consider frailty in HIV-infected adults

Source: Minor redraw of Figure 1, p. 342 of Piggott DA, Erlandson KM, Yarasheski KE. (2016). Frailty in HIV: epidemiology, biology, measurement, interventions, and research needs. *Curr HIV/AIDS Rep.* December; 13(6): 340–48.

Note

The proposed pathway is based on existing evidence derived from the general population, HIV-specific frailty literature, and emerging evidence and multi-disciplinary ideas about psychosocial and physiological inter-relationships among contributors, confounders, pathogenesis, phenotypes, and recognised outcomes or behaviours in frailty.

Androgen disorders

I will mention hormonal therapy in my discussion of interventions later in this book in Chapter 6, but androgen disorders provide some of the background. Testosterone plays key roles in regulating muscle mass and fat mass (Bhasin, 2008), and it declines with age in both men (Feldman *et al.*, 2002) and women (Davison *et al.*, 2005). Testosterone insufficiency has been shown to lead to increased visceral fat mass and decreased lean body mass (Woodhouse *et al.*, 2004) and muscle strength (O'Donnell *et al.*, 2006). In a recent prospective cohort study of community-dwelling men aged 70 years and older, lower total and free testosterone levels and higher LH (luteinising hormone) levels were associated with frailty in cross-sectional analyses (Hyde *et al.*, 2010). Moreover, treatment with testosterone can increase muscle mass while reducing visceral fat accumulation in the elderly (Allan *et al.*, 2008). Thus, age-related testosterone insufficiency may initiate the development of frailty in the elderly.

It is apparent that any relationship between androgen levels and frailty in ageing men may be modest. Most studies show weak effects of testosterone on measures of muscle mass, with weaker and less consistent effects on strength and function (O'Connell *et al.*, 2011). Prospective data from a recent study support the hypothesis that higher androgen levels may protect elderly men from worsening frailty

(Swiecicka *et al.*, 2017). However, the causal nature of these relationships requires further investigation. Whereas raised gonadotrophins in men <60 years might be an early marker of frailty, the role of oestradiol in frailty needs further clarification.

Acute care and the comprehensive geriatric assessment

Multidimensional models are important for assessing and managing older people with frailty.

The **comprehensive geriatric assessment** is widely accepted as the 'gold standard' for assessing older people living with frailty. The observations of high rates of institutionalisation in the frail older population and the inadequacy of provision for readily recognisable and remedial problems in this high-risk group led to the development of one of the cornerstones of modern geriatric care: comprehensive geriatric assessment (CGA) (Pilotto *et al.*, 2017). The concept is that the early identification of individuals at greatest risk for complications and unfavourable outcomes would enable a more adequate treatment plan and a better allocation of the resources available to the multidisciplinary team (Le Corvoisier *et al.*, 2014). CGA improves outcomes for older people in various settings, including reduced mortality or deterioration, improved cognition, improved quality of life, reduced length of stay, reduced readmission rates, reduced rates of long-term care use and reduced costs (Beswick *et al.*, 2008; Ellis *et al.*, 2011).

As illustration of 'multidisciplinary working', for example, GPs, clinical nurse specialists and geriatricians often provide clinical leadership for integrated, multidisciplinary teams which draw together professionals from right across health and social care services. Having integrated health and social care teams should ideally mean patients having faster access to services; previously, getting in touch with a social worker, district nurse, physiotherapist and occupational therapist required multiple phone calls, but now all of these services might be accessible through a single port of call. (I return to person-centred integrated care and care pathways for frailty in the final chapter, Chapter 7).

CGA emphasises problem solving, functional status and prognosis, with the aim of restoring independence and alleviating distress (Rubenstein and Rubenstein, 1991; Ellis and Langhorne, 2005).

Comprehensive geriatric assessment has been proposed as a holistic approach to meeting the needs of older patients. It is defined as 'a multidimensional interdisciplinary diagnostic process focused on determining a frail older person's medical, psychological, and functional capability in order to develop a coordinated and integrated plan for treatment and long-term follow-up' (Ellis *et al.*, 2011). CGA, indicated to explore effectively these multiple domains of health, is indeed the multidimensional and multidisciplinary tool of choice to determine the clinical profile, pathological risk, residual skills, and short- and long-term prognosis to define the personalised therapeutic and care plan of the functionally compromised and frail older individual so as to facilitate clinical decision making (Pilotto *et al.*,

2017). CGA differs from the standard medical evaluation because of its suitability for assessing frail older people with complex problems, emphasis on functional status and quality of life, use of interdisciplinary teams, and quantitative assessment scales (Suijker *et al.*, 2012). Moreover, CGA can vary in intensity from screening assessment (focused on identifying older persons' problems performed by primary care/community health workers) to thorough diagnostic assessment and management of these problems carried out by a multidisciplinary team with geriatric training and experience (e.g. Pilotto *et al.*, 2009).

The key components of the CGA are shown in Box 2.1.

BOX 2.1 KEY COMPONENTS OF COMPREHENSIVE GERIATRIC ASSESSMENT

Medical
Psychological
Functional capacity
Social circumstances
Home environment

It is recommended that organisations might wish to develop their own assessment templates and documentation; however, the domains in Table 2.1 could be included as a minimum in an effective CGA.

In addition, a multidisciplinary team should deliver the CGA. This must include as a minimum:

- a competent specialist physician in medical care of older people;
- a coordinating specialist nurse with experience;
- a senior social worker or a specialist nurse who is also a care manager with direct access to care services;
- dedicated appropriate therapists;
- the older person and their family, carers or friends.

(NHS England, 2014, p. 17)

The 'emergency department conversion rate' is increasingly recognised as a key determinant of subsequent resource use, not least because older people admitted to hospital are at high risk of adverse events, including long stays, high readmission rates and high rates of long-term care use (Conroy *et al.*, 2014). CGA screening of acute medical inpatients by a specialist team leading to early intervention improved clinical effectiveness and general hospital performance. This intervention effectively targeted a large population with small resources, and is generalisable within health systems where there are geriatric beds, multidisciplinary expertise and outpatient capacity (Harari *et al.*, 2007).

TABLE 2.1 Documenting decisions

Medical	Mental health	Functional capacity	Social circumstances	Environment
Comorbid conditions	Cognition	ADLs	Informal support	Home comfort/ facilities
Disease severity	Mood/anxiety	Gait/balance	Social network/ activities	Personal safety
Medication review (e.g. STOPP START criteria)	Fears	Activity/ exercise status	Eligibility for care resources	Use of potential use of telehealth/ telecare
Nutritional status				Transport facilities
Problem list				Accessibility of local resources

Source: adapted from www.england.nhs.uk/wp-content/uploads/2014/02/safe-comp-care.pdf, p. 17.

A recent Cochrane review entitled 'Comprehensive geriatric assessment for older adults admitted to hospital' concluded that older patients are more likely to be alive and in their own homes at follow-up if they received CGA on admission to hospital (Ellis *et al.*, 2017). There has been considerable discussion in the literature about the admission criteria for entry to geriatric care. CGA consensus conferences have supported targeting to maximise the benefit of CGA. The most common targeting criteria are a combination of age, physical disease, geriatric syndromes, impairment of functional ability and social problems (Ellis and Langhorne, 2005). These targets are often seen as methods of focusing care on those who are likely to benefit most by excluding those who are too well (functionally independent) or too sick (terminal illness and advanced dementia) (Ellis and Langhorne, 2005).

Hospitalisation is a sentinel life event for many older adults. In addition to the risk of death, around 30–40 per cent of older adults will leave hospital with a new, often persistent, disability leaving them reliant on family or needing formal care (Boyd *et al.*, 2008; Covinsky *et al.*, 2011). Recently, the Multidimensional Prognostic Index, a predictive tool of mortality based on a standardised CGA, has been developed and validated in several acute and chronic clinical conditions of hospitalised older patients (Pilotto *et al.*, 2016).

Identification of frailty

At the outset, it is worth having an overview of the development of frailty (see Figure 2.3).

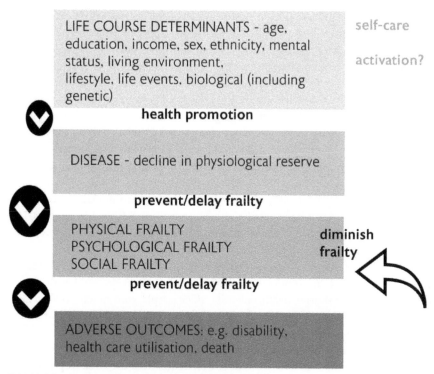

FIGURE 2.3 An integral conceptual model of frailty

Source: adapted from Figure 1, p. 620 of Gobbens RJ, van Assen MA, Luijkx KG, Schols JM. (2012). The predictive validity of the Tilburg Frailty Indicator: disability, health care utilisation, and quality of life in a population at risk. *Gerontologist*. October; 52(5): 619–31. doi:10.1093/geront/gnr135. Epub 2012 January 4.

Note
The model expresses the relationships between life-course determinants, disease or diseases (multimorbidity), frailty and adverse outcomes. The adverse outcomes in the model, which are all health-related outcomes, include disability, health care utilisation and death.

The point of identifying persons who are frail

The early recognition and timely management of frailty syndromes are important. Sometimes the terms 'screening' and 'case finding' are used interchangeably, but this is not terribly helpful. For true screening of frailty to be justified, the Wilson–Jungner criteria (1968) would have to be satisfied.[1] Increasing life expectancy of many populations in the world has raised concerns regarding possible increase of disease and disability burden, and at the same time triggered initiatives to promote healthy ageing by the adoption of healthy lifestyles to reduce the onset of common chronic diseases with age and also the onset of frailty (Woo *et al.*, 2006). The latter concept covers physical, psychological, social and environmental factors.

Commissioner and provider organisations need to decide which case finding and identification tools they will use, but it is important to have a consistent approach across all organisations involved in the care pathway. Possible further benefits to frailty case finding, at least in the older population, is providing additional risk assessment for those requiring invasive procedures (Kehler et al., 2017). For example, frailty is shown to increase one's risk for postoperative cardiac-surgical outcomes (Sepehri et al., 2014); identifying someone who is frail could lead to more conservative approaches that could help maximise a frail older adult's quality of life. On the other hand, frailty screening could lead to identifying incorrectly someone as frail who is not and might result in withholding beneficial treatments in favour of more conservative approaches (Kehler et al., 2017).

By systematically recognising frailty, we might be able to implement care processes to meet this growing societal and health problem (Muscedere et al., 2016). For example, the increasing number of older persons is one of the major threats for the sustainability of modern healthcare systems.

Clegg and colleagues (2016) have worked to develop and validate an electronic frailty index (eFI) using routinely available primary care electronic health record data. The eFI uses routine data to identify older people with mild, moderate and severe frailty, with robust predictive validity for outcomes of mortality, hospitalisation and nursing home admission. From 1 July 2017, the General Medical Services contract required practices to routinely identify moderate and severe frailty in patients aged 65 years and over.[2] Practices were required to use an appropriate tool, for example the electronic frailty index (eFI), to identify patients aged 65 and over who are living with moderate or severe frailty. For those patients identified as living with severe frailty, the diagnosis must be recorded in the patient's record. In future, there might be more objective and patient-tailored comparisons of needs and resources, potentially supporting monitoring activities aimed at the identification of apparent discrepancies (Cesari et al., 2016).

Identification of frailty can also potentially assist healthcare providers to appropriately counsel patients at a better time, and educate family members on the risks of proposed medical interventions (Lee et al., 2015; Lee et al., 2017). It is vital to know how to enrol the person with frailty in post-assessment care and support planning and associated interventions. Shropshire CCG has supported a programme to recruit and train practice-based volunteers who help connect patients with voluntary and community sector services.[3]

Measures of frailty

Perhaps most importantly, a 'test for frailty' should be quick and easy to administer, ideally utilising data that are readily available to clinicians. The sensitivity should be high enough to make the exercise worthwhile while retaining the specificity to prevent indiscriminate use of resources (Subbe and Jones, 2015). A consensus has yet to be achieved regarding the dimensions or variables that must be measured for an operational definition of frailty, or in fact how to best measure them, especially in the acute care setting. There is no agreement as to when and where these variables should be measured, the characteristics of a successful frailty assessment instrument and the organisational structures that will help facilitate it (Soong et al., 2016). Although different instruments identify closely related high-risk groups of patients, instruments are known to vary in their content validity, feasibility, and ability to predict adverse health outcomes.

To date, many different frailty instruments have been used to identify high-risk patients in the acute care setting (McIsaac et al., 2016).

> Understanding frailty, planning care, and measuring change each benefit from conceptualising frailty as a state. It is not all or none; grades of frailty make a difference. Still, many studies classify people simply as frail or non-frail. Sometimes this is useful – e.g. comparing frailty prevalence across samples. Still, important information gets lost. Many clinical decisions, sometimes including screening as well as assessment, require greater precision than frail/non-frail.
>
> *(Rockwood* et al.*, 2015, p. 545)*

The relative proliferation of 'frailty ascertainment methodologies' might potentially have benefits; for example, it could offer clinicians and researchers a selection of instruments from which to choose and facilitate the tailoring of frailty assessments to unique patients and clinical settings. However, there are also potential drawbacks. If the methodologies measure fundamentally different aspects of older adults' health or if they are differentially effective in accomplishing the goals of frailty ascertainment, then frailty-related advances and their genuine translation into effective clinical practice will be compromised (Xue et al., 2016). In elderly populations, frailty is associated with higher mortality risk. Although many frailty scores have been proposed, no single score is yet, arguably, considered the gold standard.

At the same time, the identification of a 'gold standard' measure might still be important to obtain because it represents the only way for providing the construct of a nosological entity to the often ambiguous frailty condition (Cesari et al., 2016). Major differences in the assessment of frailty exist in the clinical practice when taking care of older people. It has greatly helped to pin down frailty through objective means reflecting massive progress in translational research.

The 'frailty index' and 'frailty phenotype' are commonly quoted. Table 2.2 shows a comparison between them.

Identifying 'pre-frailty'

Pre-frailty is characterised as a modifiable intermediate state of physical frailty (Fried et al., 2001). In ageing societies, it is helpful if older individuals in the early stage of frailty (pre-frailty) are accurately diagnosed and given interventions that help prevent the progression of frailty and the need for long-term care. But it is a dangerous game to play if physicians take on the role of astrologers, and patients become dependent on accurate predictions about disease progression. One can

TABLE 2.2 Main characteristics of the frailty phenotype and the frailty index

Frailty phenotype	Frailty index
Signs, symptoms	Diseases, activities of daily living, results of a clinical evaluation
Scored robust, pre-frail or frail	Scored 0–1
Performance-based	Achievable through a comprehensive clinical assessment
Categorical variable	Continuous variable
Predefined set of criteria	Unspecified set of criteria
Frailty as a pre-disability syndrome	Frailty as an accumulation of deficits
Meaningful results potentially restricted to non-disabled older persons	Meaningful results in every individual, independently of functional status or age

Source: based on Cesari *et al.*, 2014, p.11, table 1.

only ignore the complexity of frailty at one's peril. Identifying pre-frailty is a worthy goal in itself. In a recently published study, older adults who met criteria for frailty demonstrated poorer performance in attention, verbal memory and overall global cognitive functioning compared to healthy controls. Moreover, pre frail and frail older adults had significantly worse health outcomes including greater perceived difficulty with lower and upper extremity functioning and perceived limitations in completing daily activities, suggesting the need for targeted interventions for a community that may ameliorate age-related health decline (Sleight and Holtzer, 2017). Effective interventions must be more effective in the pre-frailty than in the frailty phase. Recent work has shown that adults with intellectual and developmental disabilities experience higher rates of frailty at much earlier ages than the general population (Martin *et al.*, 2017).

Finding those who are 'pre-frail' aims to identify and target people who might benefit from more timely intervention, however.

While many experience worsening of frailty status, stability and improvement are viable goals of care. In a recent study, using multivariate logistic regression models, the authors identified the following factors as being associated with pre-frailty status: chronic constipation, occurrence of incontinence, low physical ability (unable to climb stairs), dry mouth and psychological factors (Matsushita *et al.*, 2016). On one hand, there is successful ageing or robustness when the assets largely outweigh the deficits. On the other hand, when deficits clearly prevail over the assets, disability will be the result. In between lies frailty, a precarious balance between the assets and the deficits of an individual. Although frailty is frequently regarded as a pre-disability state, it is generally agreed that frailty is reversible, and that not all frail older adults will eventually develop disabilities (Azzopardi *et al.*, 2016). However, not all pre-frail older adults progress onto frailty, and some may even return to a non-frail state, making it a meaningful and complex measure of physical health in the ageing population (Macuco *et al.*, 2012).

Notes

1 www.who.int/bulletin/volumes/86/4/07-050112/en.
2 www.nhsemployers.org/-/media/Employers/Documents/Primary-care-contracts/ GMS/Summary-of-requirements-for-frailty.pdf.
3 www.england.nhs.uk/wp-content/uploads/2016/03/releas-capcty-case-study-8-70.pdf.

References

Allan CA, Strauss BJ, Burger HG, Forbes EA, McLachlan RI. (2008). Testosterone therapy prevents gain in visceral adipose tissue and loss of skeletal muscle in nonobese aging men. *J Clin Endocrinol Metab*. 93: 139–46.

Azzopardi RV, Vermeiren S, Gorus E, Habbig AK, Petrovic M, Van Den Noortgate N, De Vriendt P, Bautmans I, Beyer I; Gerontopole Brussels Study Group. (2016). Linking frailty instruments to the international classification of functioning, disability, and health: a systematic review. *J Am Med Dir Assoc*. November 1; 17(11): 1066.e1–1066.e11. doi:10.1016/j.jamda.2016.07.023. Epub 2016 September 7.

Bagshaw SM, Stelfox HT, Johnson JA, McDermid RC, Rolfson DB, Tsuyuki RT, Ibrahim Q, Majumdar SR. (2015). Long-term association between frailty and health-related quality of life among survivors of critical illness: a prospective multicenter cohort study. *Crit Care Med*. May; 43(5): 973–82. doi:10.1097/CCM.0000000000000860.

Baltes PB, Baltes MM. (1990). *Successful aging: perspectives from the behavioral sciences*. New York: Cambridge University Press.

Beaudart C, Biver E, Reginster JY, Rizzoli R, Rolland Y, Bautmans I, Petermans J, Gillain S, Buckinx F, Van Beveren J, Jacquemain M, Italiano P, Dardenne N, Bruyere O. (2015). Development of a self administrated quality of life questionnaire for sarcopenia in elderly subjects: the SarQoL. *Age Ageing*. November; 44(6): 960–6. doi:10.1093/ageing/afv133. Epub 2015 October 3.

Beswick AD, Rees K, Dieppe P, Ayis S, Gooberman-Hill R, Horwood J, Ebrahim S. (2008). Complex interventions to improve physical function and maintain independent living in elderly people: a systematic review and meta-analysis. *Lancet*. 371: 725–35.

Bhasin S. (2008). Testicular disorders. In: Melmed S, Polonsky K, Larsen PR, Kronenberg H (eds), *Williams textbook of endocrinology*. Philadelphia: Saunders Elsevier, pp. 645–99.

Bilotta C, Bowling A, Casè A, Nicolini P, Mauri S, Castelli M, Vergani C. (2010). Dimensions and correlates of quality of life according to frailty status: a cross-sectional study on community dwelling older adults referred to an outpatient geriatric service in Italy. *Health Qual Life Outcomes*. June 8; 8: 56. doi:10.1186/1477-7525-8-56.

Blaum CS, Xue QL, Michelon E, Semba RD, Fried LP. (2005). The association between obesity and the frailty syndrome in older women: the Women's Health and Aging Studies. *J. Am. Geriatr. Soc*. 53: 927–34.

Bowling A, Stenner P. (2011). Which measure of quality of life performs best in older age? A comparison of the OPQOL, CASP-19 and WHOQOL-OLD. *J Epidemiol Community Health*. March; 65(3): 273–80. doi:10.1136/jech.2009.087668. Epub 2010 August 18.

Boxer R, Kleppinger A, Ahmad A, Annis K, Hager D, Kenny A. (2010). The 6-minute walk is associated with frailty and predicts mortality in older adults with heart failure. *Congest Heart Fail*. 16: 208–13.

Boyd CM, Landefeld CS, Counsell SR, Palmer RM, Fortinsky RH, Kresevic D, Covinsky KE. (2008). Recovery of activities of daily living in older adults after hospitalization for acute medical illness. *J Am Geriatr Soc.* 56(12): 2171–9.

Brañas F, Jiménez Z, Sánchez-Conde M, Dronda F, López-Bernaldo De Quirós JC, Pérez-Elías MJ, Miralles P, Ramírez M, Moreno A, Berenguer J, Moreno S. (2017). Frailty and physical function in older HIV-infected adults. *Age Ageing.* February 14: 1–5. doi:10.1093/ageing/afx013. [Epub ahead of print].

Brown TT, Qaqish RB. (2006). Antiretroviral therapy and the prevalence of osteopenia and osteoporosis: a meta-analytic review. *AIDS.* November 14; 20(17): 2165–74. doi: 10.1097/QAD.0b013e32801022eb.

Cacciatore F, Abete P, Mazzella F, Viati L, Della Morte D, D'Ambrosio D, Gargiulo G, Testa G, Santis D, Galizia G, Ferrara N, Rengo F. (2005). Frailty predicts long-term mortality in elderly subjects with chronic heart failure. *Eur J Clin Invest.* 35: 723–30.

Cesari M, Costa N, Hoogendijk EO, Vellas B, Canevelli M, Pérez-Zepeda MU. (2016). How the Frailty Index may support the allocation of health care resources: an example from the INCUR Study. *J Am Med Dir Assoc.* May 1; 17(5): 448–50. doi:10.1016/j.jamda.2016.02.007. Epub 2016 March 17.

Cesari M, Gambassi G, van Kan GA, Vellas B. (2014). The frailty phenotype and the frailty index: different instruments for different purposes. *Age Ageing.* January; 43(1): 10–2. doi:10.1093/ageing/aft160. Epub 2013 October 16.

Cesari M, Nobili A, Vitale G. (2016). Frailty and sarcopenia: from theory to clinical implementation and public health relevance. *Eur J Intern Med.* 35: 1–9.

Clegg A, Bates C, Young J, Ryan R, Nichols L, Ann Teale E, Mohammed MA, Parry J, Marshall T. (2016). Development and validation of an electronic frailty index using routine primary care electronic health record data. *Age Ageing.* May; 45(3): 353–60. doi:10.1093/ageing/afw039. Epub 2016 March 3.

Conroy SP, Ansari K, Williams M, Laithwaite E, Teasdale B, Dawson J, Mason S, Banerjee J. (2014). A controlled evaluation of comprehensive geriatric assessment in the emergency department: the 'Emergency Frailty Unit'. *Age Ageing.* January; 43(1): 109–14. doi:10.1093/ageing/aft087. Epub 2013 July 23.

Covinsky KE, Pierluissi E, Johnston CB. (2011). Hospitalization-associated disability: 'She was probably able to ambulate, but I'm not sure'. *JAMA.* 306(16): 1782–93.

Davison SL, Bell R, Donath S, Montalto JG, Davis SR. (2005). Androgen levels in adult females: changes with age, menopause, and oophorectomy. *J Clin Endocrinol Metab.* 90: 3847–53.

Derck JE, Thelen AE, Cron DC, Friedman JF, Gerebics AD, Englesbe MJ, Sonnenday CJ. (2015). Quality of life in liver transplant candidates: frailty is a better indicator than severity of liver disease. *Transplantation.* February; 99(2): 340–4. doi:10.1097/TP.0000000000000593.

Desquilbet L, Jacobson LP, Fried LP, Phair JP, Jamieson BD, Holloway M, Margolick JB; Multicenter AIDS Cohort Study. (2007). HIV-1 infection is associated with an earlier occurrence of a phenotype related to frailty. *J Gerontol A Biol Sci Med Sci.* November; 62(11): 1279–86.

Desquilbet L, Margolick JB, Fried LP, Phair JP, Jamieson BD, Holloway M, Jacobson LP. (2009). Relationship between a frailty-related phenotype and progressive deterioration of the immune system in HIV-infected men. *J Acquir Immune Defic Syndr.* 50: 299–306.

Dominguez-Rodriguez A, Abreu-Gonzalez P, Jimenez-Sosa A, Gonzalez J, Caballero-Estevez N, Martín-Casañas FV, Lara-Padron A, Aranda JM Jr. (2015). The impact of frailty in older patients with nonischaemic cardiomyopathy after implantation of cardiac resynchronization therapy defibrillator. *Europace.* 17: 598–602.

Ellis G, Langhorne P. (2005). Comprehensive geriatric assessment for older hospital patients. *Br Med Bull.* January 31; 71: 45–59. Print 2004.

Ellis G, Gardner M, Tsiachristas A, Langhorne P, Burke O, Harwood RH, Conroy SP, Kircher T, Somme D, Saltvedt I, Wald H, O'Neill D, Robinson D, Shepperd S. (2017). Comprehensive geriatric assessment for older adults admitted to hospital. *Cochrane Database Syst Rev.* September 12; 9: CD006211. doi:10.1002/14651858.CD006211.pub3.

Ellis G, Whitehead MA, Robinson D, O'Neill D, Langhorne P. (2011). Comprehensive geriatric assessment for older adults admitted to hospital: meta-analysis of randomised controlled trials. *BMJ.* October 27; 343: d6553. doi:10.1136/bmj.d6553.

Erlandson KM, Allshouse AA, Jankowski CM, Lee EJ, Rufner KM, Palmer BE, Wilson CC, MaWhinney S, Kohrt WM, Campbell TB. (2013). Association of functional impairment with inflammation and immune activation in HIV type 1-infected adults receiving effective antiretroviral therapy. *J Infect Dis.* 208: 249–59.

Erlandson KM, Schrack JA, Jankowski CM, Brown TT, Campbell TB. (2014). Functional impairment, disability, and frailty in adults aging with HIV infection. *Curr HIV/AIDS Rep.* 11(3): 279–90.

Feldman HA, Longcope C, Derby CA, Johannes CB, Araujo AB, Coviello AD, Bremner WJ, McKinlay JB. (2002). Age trends in the level of serum testosterone and other hormones in middle-aged men: longitudinal results from the Massachusetts male aging study. *J Clin Endocrinol Metab.* 87: 589–98.

Fried LP, Tangen CM, Walston J, Newman AB, Hirsch C, Gottdiener J, Seeman T, Tracy R, Kop WJ, Burke G, McBurnie MA (2001). Frailty in older adults evidence for a phenotype. *J Gerontol Ser A Biol Sci Med Sci.* 56(3): M146–M157.

Gabriel Z, Bowling A. (2004). Quality of life from the perspectives of older people. *Ageing and Society.* 24: 673–91.

García-Esquinas E, Graciani A, Guallar-Castillón P, López-García E, Rodríguez-Mañas L, Rodríguez-Artalejo F. (2015). Diabetes and risk of frailty and its potential mechanisms: a prospective cohort study of older adults. *J Am Med Dir Assoc.* September 1; 16(9): 748–54. doi:10.1016/j.jamda.2015.04.008. Epub 2015 May 16.

Gilhooly M, Gilhooly K, Bowling A. (2005). Quality of life: meaning and measurement. In: Walker A (ed.) *Understanding quality of life in old age.* Maidenhead, UK: Open University Press.

Gill TM, Gahbauer EA, Han L, Allore HG. (2010). Trajectories of disability in the last year of life. *N Engl J Med.* 362: 1173–80.

Gobbens RJ, van Assen MA. (2016). Psychometric properties of the Dutch WHOQOL-OLD. *Health Qual Life Outcomes.* July 15; 14(1): 103. doi:10.1186/s12955-016-0508-5.

Gobbens RJ, Schols JM, van Assen MA. (2017). Exploring the efficiency of the Tilburg Frailty Indicator: a review. *Clin Interv Aging.* October 19; 12: 1739–52. doi:10.2147/CIA.S130686. eCollection 2017.

Goldwater DS, Pinney SP. (2015). Frailty in advanced heart failure: a consequence of aging or a separate entity? *Clin Med Insights Cardiol.* July 13; 9(Suppl. 2): 39–46. doi:10.4137/CMC.S19698. eCollection 2015.

Gregersen M, Jordansen MM, Gerritsen DL. (2015). Overall Quality of Life (OQoL) questionnaire in frail elderly: a study of reproducibility and responsiveness of the Depression List (DL). *Arch Gerontol Geriatr.* January–February; 60(1): 22–7. doi:10.1016/j.archger.2014.10.012. Epub 2014 October 23.

Gustafson DR, Shi Q, Thurn M, Holman S, Minkoff H, Cohen M, Plankey MW, Havlik R, Sharma A, Gange S, Gandhi M, Milam J, Hoover D. (2016). Frailty and constellations of factors in aging HIV-infected and uninfected women: the Women's Interagency HIV Study. *J Frailty Aging.* 5(1): 43–8.

Guyatt GH, Eagle DJ, Sackett B, Willan A, Griffith L, McIlroy W, Pattersonz CJ, Turpie I. (1993). Measuring quality of life in the frail elderly. *Journal of Clinical Epidemiology*. 46: 1433–44.

Hao Q, Song X, Yang M, Rockwood K. (2016). Understanding risk in the oldest old: frailty and the metabolic syndrome in a Chinese community sample aged 90+ years. *J Nutr Heal Aging*. 20: 82–8. doi:10.1007/s12603-016-0680-7.

Harari D, Martin FC, Buttery A, O'Neill S, Hopper A. (2007). The older persons' assessment and liaison team 'OPAL': evaluation of comprehensive geriatric assessment in acute medical inpatients. *Age Ageing*. November; 36(6): 670–5. Epub 2007 July 26.

Hubbard RE, Woodhouse KW. (2010). Frailty, inflammation and the elderly. *Biogerontology*. 11(5): 635–41.

Hubbard RE, Andrew MK, Fallah N, Rockwood K. (2010). Comparison of the prognostic importance of diagnosed diabetes, co-morbidity and frailty in older people. *Diabet. Med.* 27: 603–6.

Hubbard RE, O'Mahony MS, Savva GM, Calver BL, Woodhouse KW. (2009). Inflammation and frailty measures in older people. *J Cell Mol Med*. 13: 3103–9.

Jeffery CA, Shum DW, Hubbard RE. (2013). Emerging drug therapies for frailty. *Maturitas*. January; 74(1): 21–5. doi:10.1016/j.maturitas.2012.10.010. Epub 2012 November 7.

Jha SR, Hannu MK, Chang S, Montgomery E, Harkess M, Wilhelm K, Hayward CS, Jabbour A, Spratt PM, Newton P, Davidson PM, MacDonald PS. (2016). The prevalence and prognostic significance of frailty in patients with advanced heart failure referred for heart transplantation. *Transplantation*. 100: 429–36.

Kehler DS, Ferguson T, Stammers AN, Bohm C, Arora RC, Duhamel TA, Tangri N. (2017). Prevalence of frailty in Canadians 18–79 years old in the Canadian Health Measures Survey. *BMC Geriatr*. January 21; 17(1): 28. doi:10.1186/s12877-017-0423-6.

Kojima G, Iliffe S, Morris RW, Taniguchi Y, Kendrick D, Skelton DA, Masud T, Bowling A. (2016). Frailty predicts trajectories of quality of life over time among British community-dwelling older people. *Qual Life Res*. July; 25(7): 1743–50. doi:10.1007/s11136-015-1213-2. Epub 2016 January 9.

Le Corvoisier P, Bastuji-Garin S, Renaud B, Mahe I, Bergmann JF, Perchet H, Paillaud E, Mottier D, Montagne O. (2014). Functional status and co-morbidities are associated with in-hospital mortality among older patients with acute decompensated heart failure: a multicentre prospective cohort study. *Age Ageing*. 43(Suppl. 2): ii1–ii26.

Lee L, Heckman G, Molnar FJ. (2015). Frailty: identifying elderly patients at high risk of poor outcomes. *Can Fam Physician*. 61: 227–31.

Lee L, Patel T, Hillier LM, Maulkhan N, Slonim K, Costa A. (2017). Identifying frailty in primary care: a systematic review. *Geriatr Gerontol Int*. April 12. doi:10.1111/ggi.12955. [Epub ahead of print].

Lisiak M, Uchmanowicz I, Wontor R. (2016). Frailty and quality of life in elderly patients with acute coronary syndrome. *Clin Interv Aging*. May 5; 11: 553–62. doi:10.2147/CIA.S99842. eCollection 2016.

Macuco CRM, Batistoni SST, Lopes A, Cachioni M. (2012). Mini-mental state examination performance in frail, pre-frail, and non-frail community dwelling older adults in Ermelino Matarazzo, São Paulo, Brazil. *International Psychogeriatrics*. 24(11): 1725–31.

Mansur HN, Colugnati FA, Grincenkov FR, Bastos MG. (2014). Frailty and quality of life: a cross-sectional study of Brazilian patients with pre-dialysis chronic kidney disease. *Health Qual Life Outcomes*. February 28; 12: 27. doi:10.1186/1477-7525-12-27.

Margolick J, Martinez-Maza O, Jacobson L, Lopez J, Li X, Phair J, Bream JH, Koletar SL. (2013). *Frailty and circulating markers of inflammation in HIVR and HIV – men in the multicenter AIDS Cohort Study*. 20th Conference on Retroviruses and Opportunistic Infections, Atlanta, Georgia, U.S.

Martin L, McKenzie K, Ouellette-Kuntz H. (2017). Once frail, always frail? Frailty transitions in home care users with intellectual and developmental disabilities. *Geriatr Gerontol Int.* December 7. doi:10.1111/ggi.13214. [Epub ahead of print].

Matsushita E, Okada K, Ito Y, Satake S, Shiraishi N, Hirose T, Kuzuya M. (2016). Characteristics of physical prefrailty among Japanese healthy older adults. *Geriatr Gerontol Int.* December 9. doi:10.1111/ggi.12935. [Epub ahead of print].

McAlister FA, Lethebe BC, Lambe C, Williamson T, Lowerison M. (2018). Control of glycemia and blood pressure in British adults with diabetes mellitus and subsequent therapy choices: a comparison across health states. *Cardiovasc Diabetol.* February 12; 17(1): 27. doi:10.1186/s12933-018-0673-4.

McDonagh J, Ferguson C, Newton PJ. (2018). Frailty assessment in heart failure: an overview of the multi-domain approach. *Curr Heart Fail Rep.* January 20. doi:10.1007/s11897-018-0373-0. [Epub ahead of print].

McDonagh J, Martin L, Ferguson C, Jha SR, Macdonald PS, Davidson PM, Newton PJ. (2017). Frailty assessment instruments in heart failure: a systematic review. *Eur J Cardiovasc Nurs.* May 1. doi: 10.1177/1474515117708888. [Epub ahead of print].

McIsaac DI, Taljaard M, Bryson GL, Beaule PE, Gagne S, Hamilton G, Hladkowicz E, Huang A, Joanisse J, Lavallée LT, Moloo H, Thavorn K, van Walraven C, Yang H, Forster AJ. (2016). Comparative assessment of two frailty instruments for risk-stratification in elderly surgical patients: study protocol for a prospective cohort study. *BMC Anesthesiol.* Nov 14; 16(1): 111.

Montero-Odasso M, Schapira M, Soriano ER, Varela M, Kaplan R, Camera LA, Mayorga LM. (2005). Gait velocity as a single predictor of adverse events in healthy seniors aged 75 years and older. *J Gerontol A Biol Sci Med Sci.* 60(10): 1304–9.

Muscedere J, Andrew MK, Bagshaw SM, Estabrooks C, Hogan D, Holroyd-Leduc J, Howlett S, Lahey W, Maxwell C, McNally M, Moorhouse P, Rockwood K, Rolfson D, Sinha S, Tholl B; Canadian Frailty Network (CFN). (2016). Screening for frailty in Canada's health care system: a time for action. *Can J Aging.* September; 35(3): 281–97. doi:10.1017/S0714980816000301. Epub 2016 May 23.

NHS England. (2014) *Safe, compassionate care for frail older people using an integrated care pathway: practical guidance for commissioners, providers and nursing, medical and allied health professional leaders.* www.england.nhs.uk/wp-content/uploads/2014/02/safe-comp-care.pdf.

O'Donnell AB, Travison TG, Harris SS, Tenover JL, McKinlay JB. (2006). Testosterone, dehydroepiandrosterone, and physical performance in older men: results from the Massachusetts Male Aging Study. *J Clin Endocrinol Metab.* 91: 425–31.

Pathai S, Gilbert C, Weiss HA, Cook C, Wood R, Bekker L-G, Lawn SD. (2013). Frailty in HIV-infected adults in South Africa. *J Acquir Immune Defic Syndr.* 62: 43–51.

Petit N, Enel P, Ravaux I, Darque A, Baumstarck K, Bregigeon S, Retornaz 8; Visage group. (2018). Frail and pre-frail phenotype is associated with pain in older HIV-infected patients. *Medicine* (Baltimore). February; 97(6): e9852. doi:10.1097/MD.0000000000009852.

Pilotto A, Addante F, D'Onofrio G, Sancarlo D, Ferrucci L. (2009). The Comprehensive Geriatric Assessment and the multidimensional approach: a new look at the older patient with gastroenterological disorders. *Best Pract Res Clin Gastroenterol.* 23(6): 829–37. doi:10.1016/j.bpg.2009.10.001.

Pilotto A, Cella A, Pilotto A, Daragjati J, Veronese N, Musacchio C, Mello AM, Logroscino G, Padovani A, Prete C, Panza F. (2017). Three decades of comprehensive geriatric assessment: evidence coming from different healthcare settings and specific clinical conditions. *J Am Med Dir Assoc.* February 1; 18(2): 192.e1–192.e11. doi:10.1016/j.jamda.2016.11.004. Epub 2016 December 31.

Pilotto A, Sancarlo D, Pellegrini F, Rengo F, Marchionni N, Volpato S, Ferrucci L; FIRI-SIGG Study Group. (2016). The Multidimensional Prognostic Index predicts in-hospital length of stay in older patients: a multicentre prospective study. *Age Ageing*. January; 45(1): 90–6. doi: 10.1093/ageing/afv167.

Provencher V, Sirois MJ, Émond M, Perry JJ, Daoust R, Lee JS, Griffith LE, Batomen Kuimi BL, Despeignes LR, Wilding L, Allain-Boulé N, Lebon J; Canadian Emergency Team Initiative on Mobility in Aging. (2016). Frail older adults with minor fractures show lower health-related quality of life (SF-12) scores up to six months following emergency department discharge. *Health Qual Life Outcomes*. March 8; 14: 40. doi:10.1186/s12955-016-0441-7.

Rockwood K, Theou O, Mitnitski A. (2015). What are frailty instruments for? *Age Ageing*. July; 44(4): 545–7. doi:10.1093/ageing/afv043. Epub 2015 March 29.

Rubenstein LZ, Rubenstein LV. (1991). Multidimensional assessment of elderly patients. *Adv Intern Med*. 36: 81–108.

Scuteri A, Najjar SS, Morrell CH, Lakatta EG. (2005). The metabolic syndrome in older individuals: prevalence and prediction of cardiovascular events: the cardiovascular health study. *Diabetes Care*. 28: 882–7.

Sepehri A, Beggs T, Hassan A, Rigatto C, Shaw-Daigle C, Tangri N, Arora RC. (2014). The impact of frailty on outcomes after cardiac surgery: a systematic review. *J Thorac Cardiovasc Surg*. December; 148(6): 3110–7. doi:10.1016/j.jtcvs.2014.07.087. Epub 2014 August 7.

Shlipak MG, Fried LF, Crump C, Bleyer AJ, Manolio TA, Tracy RP, Furberg CD, Psaty BM. (2003). Elevations of inflammatory andprocoagulant biomarkers in elderly persons with renal insufficiency. *Circulation*. 107(1): 87–92.

Sleight C, Holtzer R. (2017). Differential associations of functional and cognitive health outcomes with pre-frailty and frailty states in community-dwelling older adults. *J Health Psychol*. December 1. doi:10.1177/1359105317745964. [Epub ahead of print].

Soong JT, Poots AJ, Bell D. (2016). Finding consensus on frailty assessment in acute care through Delphi method. *BMJ Open*. October 14; 6(10): e012904. doi:10.1136/bmjopen-2016-012904.

Stanley TL, Grinspoon SK. (2012). Body composition and metabolic changes in HIV-infected patients. *J Infect Dis*. 205(Suppl. 3): 383–90.

Subbe CP, Jones S. (2015). Predicting speed at traffic lights: the problem with static assessments of frailty. *Age Ageing*. March; 44(2): 180–1. doi:10.1093/ageing/afu204. Epub 2015 January 14.

Suijker JJ, Buurman BM, ter Riet G, van Rijn M, de Haan RJ, de Rooij SE, Moll van Charante EP. (2012). Comprehensive geriatric assessment, multifactorial interventions and nurse-led care coordination to prevent functional decline in community-dwelling older persons: protocol of a cluster randomized trial. *BMC Health Serv Res*. April 1; 12: 85. doi:10.1186/1472-6963-12-85.

Swiecicka A, Eendebak RJAH, Lunt M, O'Neill TW, Bartfai G, Casanueva FF, Forti G, Giwercman A, Han TS, Slowikowska-Hilczer J, Lean MEJ, Pendleton N, Punab M, Vanderschueren D, Huhtaniemi IT, Wu FCW, Rutter MK; EMAS study group. (2017). Reproductive hormone levels predict changes in frailty status in community-dwelling older men: European Male Ageing Study prospective data. *J Clin Endocrinol Metab*. November 24. doi:10.1210/jc.2017-01172. [Epub ahead of print].

Terzian AS, Holman S, Nathwani N, Robison E, Weber K, Young M, Greenblatt RM, Gange SJ. (2009). Factors associated with preclinical disability and frailty among HIV-infected and HIV-uninfected women in the era of cART. *J Womens Health*. 18: 1965–74.

Van Malderen L, Mets T, Gorus E. (2013). Interventions to enhance the Quality of Life of older people in residential long-term care: a systematic review. *Ageing Res Rev.* January; 12(1): 141–50. doi:10.1016/j.arr.2012.03.007. Epub 2012 April 6.

Veronese N, Stubbs B, Fontana L, Trevisan C, Bolzetta F, De Rui M, Sartori L, Musacchio E, Zambon S, Maggi S, Perissinotto E, Corti MC, Crepaldi G, Manzato E, Sergi G. (2016). Frailty is associated with an increased risk of incident type 2 diabetes in the elderly. *J Am Med Dir Assoc.* October 1; 17(10): 902–7. doi:10.1016/j.jamda.2016.04.021. Epub 2016 June 7.

Viscogliosi, G. (2016). The metabolic syndrome: a risk factor for the frailty syndrome? *J. Am. Med. Dir. Assoc.* 17: 364–6.

Walker SR, Gill K, Macdonald K, Komenda P, Rigatto C, Sood MM, Bohm CJ, Storsley LJ, Tangri N. (2013). Association of frailty and physical function in patients with non-dialysis CKD: a systematic review. *BMC Nephrol.* 22(14): 228. doi:10.1186/1471-2369-14-228.

Walston J, McBurnie MA, Newman A, Tracy RP, Kop WJ, Hirsch CH, Gottdiener J, Fried LP. (2002). Frailty and activation of the inflammation and coagulation systems with and without clinical comorbidities: results from the Cardiovascular Health Study. *Arch Intern Med.* 162(20): 2333–41.

Wang J, Ruotsalainen S, Moilanen L, Lepisto P, Laakso M, Kuusisto J. (2007). The metabolic syndrome predicts cardiovascular mortality: a 13-year follow-up study in elderly non-diabetic. *Finns. Eur. Heart J.* 28: 857–64.

WHO (World Health Organization). (1995). Quality of Life assessment (WHOQOL): position paper from the World Health Organization. *Soc Sci Med.* November; 41(10): 1403–9.

Won CW, Kim S. (2016). Use of frailty in deciding clinical treatment goals for chronic disease in elderly patients in the community. *J Am Med Dir Assoc.* November 1; 17(11): 967–9. doi:10.1016/j.jamda.2016.07.019.

Woo J, Goggins W, Sham A, Ho SC. (2006). Public health significance of the frailty index. *Disabil Rehabil.* April 30; 28(8): 515–21.

Woodhouse LJ, Gupta N, Bhasin M, Singh AB, Ross R, Phillips J, Bhasin S. (2004). Dose-dependent effects of testosterone on regional adipose tissue distribution in healthy young men. *J Clin Endocrinol Metab.* 89: 718–26.

Woods NF, LaCroix AZ, Gray SL, Aragaki A, Cochrane BB, Brunner RL, Masaki K, Murray A, Newman AB. (2005). Frailty: emergence and consequences in women aged 65 and older in the Women's Health Initiative Observational Study (WHI-OS). *J Am Geriatr Soc.* 53(8): 1321–30.

Xue QL, Tian J, Fried LP, Kalyani RR, Varadhan R, Walston JD, Bandeen-Roche K. (2016). Physical frailty assessment in older women: can simplification be achieved without loss of syndrome measurement validity? *Am J Epidemiol.* June 1; 183(11): 1037–44. doi:10.1093/aje/kwv272. Epub 2016 May 5.

Yanase T, Yanagita I, Muta K, Nawata H. (2017). Frailty in elderly diabetes patients. *Endocr J.* December 14. doi:10.1507/endocrj.EJ17-0390. [Epub ahead of print].

Zachariae B, Bech, P. (2008). Livskvalitet som begreb [Quality of life concept; in Danish]. *Ugeskrift for Laeger.* 170: 821–5.

3

EVIDENCE-BASED PRACTICE IN FRAILTY

Falls and activity

Aim

In this chapter, I'd like to look at some of the evidence surrounding the falls and immobility frailty syndromes. I will argue that a more 'holistic' view of intervention is perhaps required, rather than a strictly medical one, including addressing the factors that surround impairments and disability – such as fear of falling or activity avoidance.

Introduction to frailty and fractures

There are currently unacceptably wide variations in the delivery of clinical care to older people presenting with a **hip fracture**. Of concern are the long lengths of time in A&E for many patients and the low level of routine access to preoperative medical assessment. It is hoped that the launch of joint initiatives between the British Orthopaedic Association and the British Geriatric Society aimed at delivering service improvements in this area should lead to improved outcomes (Youde *et al.*, 2009). Patients tend to experience complications, decrement of functional ability, institutionalisation and death after surgery more frequently than their younger counterparts because of their unique physiological vulnerability. Preoperative geriatric assessment markers for frailty, disability, comorbidity, biochemical marker including haemoglobin and albumin, and frailty index are known to predict adverse outcomes in older surgical or trauma patients (Choi *et al.*, 2017).

Most older people who fracture a hip are frail, have comorbidities and show a functional deterioration that is typical of geriatric patients (Auais *et al.*, 2013). After a fracture, both short-term and long-term outlooks for patients are generally poor, with increased one-year mortality (Bentler *et al.*, 2009). People who suffer a hip fracture are frailer than their age-matched peers, and hip fractures are strongly linked with causes and consequences of frailty such as osteoporosis, falls, low body mass index, polypharmacy and cognitive impairment (Krishnan *et al.*, 2014). Limited evidence for the change of frailty before and after some non-fatal adverse health events is available. Moreover, whether and to what extent the FI (frailty index) change can predict the following adverse outcomes requires further exploration (Li *et al.*, 2016). There is evidence that women have a higher likelihood of falls than men (e.g. Wei and Hester, 2014).

Non-hip fracture is associated with an almost three-fold increase in the risk of a subsequent hip fracture within the next 2.5 years in frail elderly patients compared with frail individuals without a fracture (Chen *et al.*, 2011). An increase in the rate of falling may reflect greater frailty and increased risk of fracture when a fall occurs (Schwartz *et al.*, 2005). Frailty might reflect a loss of functional homeostasis, which results in a reduced ability to withstand or compensate for illness without a loss of function. For example, an 80-year-old person is less likely than a younger person to regain pre-existing functional capacity after a hip fracture, and subsequent events could lead to progressive disability and dependence (Boots *et al.*, 2013). Moderate frailty may be related to risk of future health outcomes. The intermediate stage between no frailty and frailty (pre-frailty) may also be associated directly with risk of falls, fracture and disability. In an indirect manner, pre-frailty may increase risk of these outcomes through increasing the risk of becoming frail, but pre-frailty has been less consistently associated with health outcomes than frailty (Tom *et al.*, 2013).

Osteoporosis and osteoarthritis

Osteoporosis is a skeletal disease that reduces bone density and increases the risk of fracture (Szulc and Bouxsein, 2010). Osteoporosis is a systemic skeletal disease characterised by low bone mass and microarchitectural deterioration of bone tissue that leads to increased bone fragility and a consequent increase in fracture risk (NIH Consensus Development Panel on Osteoporosis Prevention, Diagnosis, and Therapy, 2001). Osteoporosis can occur without a known underlying cause, and is diagnosed in clinical practice by the presence of a fragility fracture or using bone mineral density (BMD) criteria. The BMD criteria were developed by the WHO on the basis of epidemiological data that describe the normal distribution of BMD in a reference population comprising healthy young adults (Writing Group for the ISCD Position Development Conference, 2004). Recently, there is an increasing body of evidence that the trabecular bone score (TBS), a surrogate of bone microarchitecture extracted from spine DXA, could play an important role in the management of patients with osteoporosis or at risk of fracture (Hans *et al.*, 2017).

Fractures in people with osteoporosis are often low trauma in origin (National Osteoporosis Guidelines Group 2014, Scottish Intercollegiate Guidelines 142 (SIGN) 2015[1]). The World Health Organization defines 'Low Trauma Fracture' (LTF) as one that results from 'forces equivalent to a fall from a standing height or less, or trauma that in a healthy individual would not give rise to fracture' (Kanis, 2007, p. 13). Incidence increases with age and, given the expansion in the ageing population worldwide, the health burden of osteoporosis is predicted to be a major global problem by 2050 (Cooper, 1992). Whereas osteoporosis is a disease resulting from disordered bone remodelling and is diagnosed using Dual Energy X-ray scanning (DEXA), frailty describes a phenomenon that is multifactorial.

Osteoporosis and frailty can co-occur leading to increased risk of fracture in the ageing population and there can be an interplay of contributing factors such as reduced mobility due to osteoarthritis, obesity and/or poor nutrition (Rizzoli *et al.*, 2014). It is well accepted that ageing is an important contributing factor to the development of **osteoarthritis**. Osteoarthritis may affect one or many joints in the same individual and represents a major cause of morbidity, disability and social isolation. This is particularly so when the main weight-bearing joints, such as the hip and knee are involved, as this may lead directly to reduced mobility (Guccione, 1997). Also, using data from the Multicenter Osteoarthritis Study and Osteoarthritis Initiative, Misra and colleagues (2015) reported that knee osteoarthritis is associated with greater prevalence and risk of developing frailty. Understanding the mechanisms linking these two common conditions of older adults would aid in identifying novel targets for treatment or prevention of frailty.

The mechanisms responsible appear to be multifactorial (see Figure 3.1), and may include an age-related pro-inflammatory state that has been termed

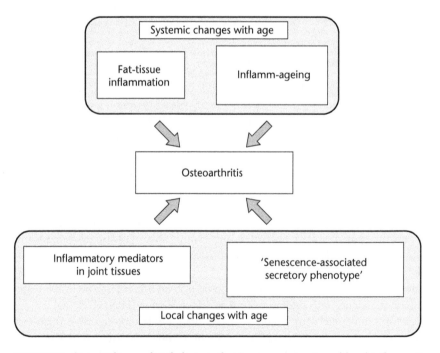

FIGURE 3.1 Potential age-related changes that increase systemic and local inflammation and promote the development of OA

Source: redrawn from Figure 1, p. 1967 of Greene MA, Loeser RF. (2015). Aging-related inflammation in osteoarthritis. *Osteoarthritis Cartilage*. November; 23(11): 1966–71. doi:10.1016/j.joca.2015.01.008.

'inflamm-ageing'. Age-related inflammation can be both systemic and local. Systemic inflammation can be promoted by ageing changes in adipose tissue that result in increased production of cytokines such as interleukin (IL)-6 and tumor necrosis factor-α (TNF-α). Numerous studies have shown an age-related increase in blood levels of IL-6 that has been associated with decreased physical function and frailty. Importantly, higher levels of IL-6 have been associated with an increased risk of knee osteoarthritis progression.

Lower levels of circulating 25-hydroxyvitamin D (25(OH)D) and frailty are increasingly common with advancing age. Several previous studies have reported that frailty independently predicts risks of adverse health outcomes including incident disability, falls, fractures and mortality (Ensrud et al., 2010). Previous cross-sectional studies have suggested that older adults with lower 25(OH)D levels are more likely to be classified as frail than not frail (Michelon et al., 2006; Puts et al., 2005). Inconsistencies between the findings of studies examining the association between 25(OH)D level and frailty status may in part be explained by differences in study populations, sample size, methods to measure 25(OH)D, cut points used to define 25(OH)D status, definitions of frailty syndrome or adequacy of adjustment for potential confounders (Ensrud et al., 2010).

The effects of vitamin D should not be underestimated.

Falls

> Falls in advanced age breaks not only bones, but also self-esteem, confidence and activity.
>
> *(Runge, 1998)*

Public Health England published in February 2018 a document entitled 'A structured literature review to identify cost-effective interventions to prevent falls in older people living in the community', reflecting the importance of serious outcomes of falls, including fracture, other injury, pain, impaired function, loss of confidence in carrying out everyday activities, loss of independence and autonomy, and even death.[2] Arguably, persons who are frail and who are at risk of falling should have a home safety evaluation. The assessment, which takes about an hour, is done by a professional with expertise in home safety, who looks for loose rugs and other hazards and suggests ways to correct them, and who can provide specific advice and guidance on changing or adapting the physical and social environment to ensure physical safety, comfort and emotional security.

Falls have been described as one of the 'Geriatric Giants' (Healey et al., 2004). They account for the greatest number (33 per cent) of adverse event reports to the National Reporting and Learning System in the UK, with 94 per cent occurring in acute inpatient facilities (Healey et al., 2008). Falls and frailty share many significant characteristics. Both are important health issues that affect older people, increase with increasing patient age and are multifactorial phenomena associated with adverse health outcomes (Nowak and Hubbard, 2009). In the Royal College of

Physicians' report (2017) 'National audit of inpatient falls: audit report' for 2017, there were three key indicators that improved significantly, albeit minimally, between the 2015 and 2017 rounds of the audit. These were: measurement of lying and standing blood pressure (from 16 to 19 per cent), delirium assessment (from 37 to 40 per cent) and mobility aid in reach (from 68 to 72 per cent). However, these rates leave considerable room for improvement in most trusts. The report concluded that there has been highly variable progress on falls prevention activities and, nationally overall, minimal progress has been made.

Falls is an important frailty syndrome, so it is important that it can be prevented. The causes of falls are multifactorial; see Figure 3.2.

Frailty is a major predictor of falls; frailty is also recognised as a risk factor for falls (Fang *et al.*, 2012. Main features of frailty include weakness, as well as balance and gait problems, all of which predispose older people to falling (Clegg *et al.*, 2013). Reliably characterising fall risk and frailty in a clinical setting has been challenging. A tool such as Stopping Elderly Accidents, Death and Injuries (STEADI) may have potential to reduce future falls by nearly 25 per cent, but there is a lack of data on its use in healthcare practice settings (Crow *et al.*, 2018).

Falls-related injuries in nursing homes have a major impact on the quality of life in later adulthood and there is a relative paucity of studies on falling and fall prevention from the older person's perspective. It is important to identify how older

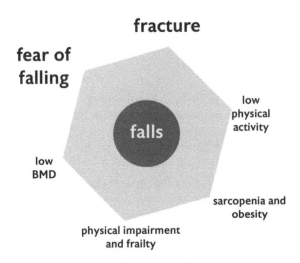

FIGURE 3.2 The multifactorial causes of falls

Source: adapted from Figure 1, p. 344 of Erlandson KM, Guaraldi G, Falutz J. (2016). More than osteoporosis: age-specific issues in bone health. *Curr Opin HIV AIDS*. May; 11(3): 343–50. doi:10.1097/COH.0000000000000258.

Note
Falls are affected by adiposity, sarcopenia, physical function impairment and low physical activity; a fall can also result in many of these same factors, leading to further physical function impairment, fear of falling and subsequent fracture.

TABLE 3.1 Identification of themes on the perception of falls

Highlighted sentences and phrases	Interpretive process (main theme)
'I was out for the count banged my head on the wall and then on the floor. I have banged my head so many times.'	An interesting subject with elements of drama (Stories of courage and endurance)
'I believe that I will get better day by day, you have to be optimistic, can't be negative.'	Externalising the problem
'I try to be independent but I don't find the roller walker easy to use. I have cushioned that handle and I try to practice.'	Being optimistic and dealing with their ailments (Meaningful activities)

Source: adapted from Clancy et al., 2015.

persons perceive falling, however. Some themes have been identified successfully from a well conducted study (see Table 3.1).

The 'fear of falling'

Most studies on **the fear of falling** (FOF) use self-efficacy related to falls as the underlying concept of explanatory models. Such concepts represent a skill set, motivation and confidence, which are essential elements in an elderly person's perceived ability to prevent falls (for example, for a wider discussion on behaviour, see Bandura, 1982). Perceived self-efficacy is an important prerequisite for successful self-management (Freund et al., 2013). The concept is theoretically and empirically well founded (Barlow et al., 2005) and was originally developed by Bandura in the 1970s. Self-efficacy is enhanced when patients succeed in solving patient-identified problems. Based on improved self-efficacy patients can regain control of their own lives, gaining new confidence in their ability to perform a task, hence increasing self-management (Bodenheimer et al., 2002). Both falls and fear of falling can substantially reduce quality of life and independence, and so contribute to the placement of an elderly person into institutional care (Lord, 1994). A recent investigation has demonstrated that FOF is associated with onset of functional disability over a two-year period in a diverse community-based population (Auais et al., 2017). The impact of FOF on this population is statistically and clinically important and is associated with a large increase in the risk of developing incident disability. Future studies should investigate potential mediators in the longitudinal relationship, and should provide further evidence for interventions to prevent and treat FOF by targeting it directly and/or targeting relevant modifiable risk factors.

Patil and colleagues (2014) found that concern about falling was highly prevalent in their sample of community-living older women. A perceived poor quality of life and health and mobility constraints contributed independently to the difference between high and low concern of falling. In a broader clinical perspective, knowledge of these associations may help in developing interventions to reduce fear of falling and activity avoidance in old age. The study by Seematter-Bagnoud and colleagues (2010) shows the existence of a relationship between fear of falling and frailty, and suggests that it is potentially mediated by falls history, but remains – at least partially – independent of gait performance. FOF and falls interact with each other, i.e. in older adults with a previous fall history, the prevalence of FOF ranges between 29 and 92 per cent; in people without a previous fall history, the rate is between 12 and 65 per cent (Murphy et al., 2002).

Fear of falling is undeniably a major health problem among community-dwelling older adults that may contribute to avoidance of activities that they are capable of performing. Community-dwelling elderly people have described FOF as a negative experience, often linked to fear of incapacitation, loss of independence and the prospect of having to move to a care facility (Lee et al., 2008). Around 25 to 85 per cent of older adults report FoF; among these, 20 to 55 per cent curtail their physical activities as a result of their concerns (Murphy et al., 2003). Fear of falling is not exclusive to very old people who have a history of falls, as up to 50 per cent of persons reporting fear of falling do not have a fall history (Scheffer et al., 2008). The prevalence of fear of falling varies between 12 and 65 per cent for independent elderly individuals without a history of falls, and 29 and 92 per cent in those with a history of falls (Legters, 2002).

Table 3.2 presents the prevalence of fear of falling according to the clinical and functional variables.

Many elderly people can underestimate or overestimate their risk of falling. Measures of both physiological and perceived fall risk should be included in fall risk assessments to allow tailoring of interventions for preventing falls in elderly people (Delbaere et al., 2010). Interestingly, it appears that cognitive impairment is significantly associated with the absence of FoF in community-dwelling frail older adults. In addition, among frail older adults, the score on the attention and calculation subsection of the MMSE was positively associated with the presence of FoF (Shirooka et al., 2017). Tinetti and Powell (1993) define fear of falling as a constant concern about falling that limits the performance of activities of daily living (ADL). It was initially described as a result of falls, and is the central component of post-fall syndrome (Murphy and Isaacs, 1982). It is also reported in individuals with *no history* of falls (Legters, 2002; Hadjistavropoulos et al., 2011).

Affective status or depression can adversely affect recovery after hip fracture as well. Depression can augment behavioural symptoms of cognitive impairment and may affect the capacity to participate in rehabilitation (Beaupre et al., 2013). There is generally mounting evidence that positive affect, defined as emotional contentment and happiness, has benefits for physical and psychological health. It is associated with greater independence in ADLs; faster walking speed; and lower incidence of mortality, stroke and frailty in community-dwelling elderly adults (Park-Lee et al., 2009). Since the identification of the '**post-fall syndrome**' in the 1980s (Murphy and Isaacs, 1982), FOF has gained recognition as a health problem in the elderly (Letgers, 2002).

TABLE 3.2 Expanded prevalence of fear of falling according to clinical and functional characteristics (Rio de Janeiro Study, 2010)

Variables	n	(%)	Prevalence of fear of falling (%)	P
History of falls				
No falls	531	(71.6)	44.1	
1–2 falls	175	(23.6)	66.7	★
Comorbidities				
0–1	300	(40.4)	40.5	
2–3	358	(48.2)	55.1	★
No. medications				
0–3	311	(41.9)	39.8	
4–6	261	(35.2)	53.4	★
Hearing impairment				
No	560	(75.5)	47.5	
Yes	182	(24.5)	62.9	★
Visual impairment				
No	497	(67.0)	46.6	
Yes	245	(33.0)	61	★
Functional dependency (ADL)				
No	601	(81.0)	46.1	
Yes	141	(19.0)	64.7	★
Self-rated health				
Very good/good	416	(56.1)	40.5	
Fair	291	(39.2)	62.6	★
Poor/very poor	35	(4.7)	88.4	

Source: adapted from Malini *et al.*, 2016.

Note
★$P < 0.001$; ADL, activities of daily living.

Management of the 'fear of falling'

Research on interventions that aim to reduce fear of falling and increase activity in older adults is needed (Halvarsson *et al.*, 2011; Zijlstra, 2007; Zijlstra *et al.*, 2007). Multicomponent interventions that combine cognitive behaviour therapy with balance training, exercise and home safety assessments may be most effective at reducing fall rate and fear of falling in community-dwelling older adults (Freiberger *et al.*, 2006; Gillespie *et al.*, 2012; Zijlstra *et al.*, 2007). Furthermore, home-based interventions are warranted to reach those individuals who are most fearful and thus may benefit the most from treatment (Tennstedt *et al.*, 1998).

The cognitive–behavioural interrelationship of a situation or practical problem (falls, declining mobility, social isolation), altered thinking and emotion, altered physical symptoms with behavioural change, and activity reduction and avoidance appears to form the crux of fear of falling, and therefore may offer the hope of a realistic interventional option (Williams, 2002). Previous studies are hampered by poor documentation of power calculations, high dropout rates from intervention groups, group rather than individual therapy, lack of recording of quality of life measures and the absence of health-economic analysis (Parry *et al.*, 2016). Behavioural change is of substantial importance to improve people's live with frailty. As rates of lifestyle-related chronic diseases and associated costs continue to rise in the United States, there has been an increasing focus on identifying successful behavioural interventions to help patients prevent and manage disease (Simmons and Wolever, 2013). Two frequently cited behavioural approaches include health coaching and motivational interviewing.

It appears that **avoidance of activities because of FOF** increases with the degree of FOF. FOF decreases levels of mobility, and disability might lead to social isolation and despair. In the years to come, the prevalence of hip fracture is expected to increase with more cost to society. Consequently, focus on FOF and efforts to prevent avoidance of activities in the elderly after a hip fracture may be important. However, there is a need for longitudinal studies on the consequences of FOF and prevention or reduction of FOF in patients recovering from a hip fracture (Jellesmark *et al.*, 2012). Fear of falling is one of the most common fears among community-dwelling older people and is as serious a health problem as falls themselves. Personalised assessment and education for falls prevention is very resource intensive, and it has therefore been argued that it is only reliably cost-effective for those most at risk of falling due to older age or medical risk factors (Chang *et al.*, 2004; Gillespie, 2004; Kannus *et al.*, 2005).

Various systematic reviews have focused on the benefits of interventions to reduce FOF in older people living in the community (Kendrick *et al.*, 2014; Zijlstra *et al.*, 2007). A recent systematic review found 12 high-quality randomised controlled trials (RCTs) reporting effects on fear of falling in such studies, but only one primarily aimed at reducing fear of falling (Austin *et al.*, 2007). The interventions were conducted across a variety of settings, but home-based exercise, community tai chi and home-based multifactorial interventions all improved fear of falling (Zijlstra *et al.*, 2007), though a recent geriatric outpatient-based multifactorial intervention study found no such benefit (BonnerupVind *et al.*, 2010).

Activity restriction and avoidance

Thinking about how people who are frail function at home, in their own living environment, is pivotal, and should not be dismissed as unimportant for the duration of a hospital admission. When people withdraw from activities of daily living (ADL) and outdoor social contact, they become more susceptible to the negative effects of social isolation and physical inactivity. **Activity avoidance** also increases loss of muscle strength and postural control. Delbaere and colleagues (2004) found substantial evidence for the association between avoidance of feared activities on the one hand and physical performance, muscle strength and postural performance on the other hand. These associations were most pronounced for mobility activities such as walking and reaching, and less pronounced for ADL and social activities. Mobility disability is a precursor of more than half of end-stage disability in older adults and it is more common among women (Fried et al., 2000; Zunzunegui et al., 2015). It is usually defined as the self-reported difficulty to walk 400 m without resting or to climb a flight of stairs without support (Gill et al., 2006). Activity restriction due to fear of falling when present in excessive level may provide loss of independence for reducing the social interaction, which in turn leads to physical inactivity and reduced quality of life (Arfken et al., 1994; Murphy et al., 2002). Activity restriction is a predictor of falls, possibly because of the decline of muscle function, physical '**deconditioning**', balance and gait disorders (Rochat et al., 2010). The importance and benefits of embracing 'positive risk', e.g. mobilisation/ falls, are seen clearly in the #endPJparalysis initiative.

'Preventive home visits' may also provide a useful opportunity for education about prevention of falls (see Box 3.1).

BOX 3.1 DISCUSSION OF AREAS IN 'PREVENTIVE HOME VISIT INTERVENTIONS'

Common health problems connected with advancing age
How to prevent identified fall risks and how to continue be active; assessment of the fall prevention checklist
A basic home exercise programme including balance exercises
Activities provided by the community, for instance local meeting places, activities run by local associations, physical training, walking groups, and possibility of receiving or providing volunteer interventions
Walking groups, a short introduction to computer skills, and other activities
Public transportation, buses adapted for older adults and mobility service for the disabled
Possibility to meet a pharmacist for counselling on medicines

Reference: Zidén et al., 2014.

Although some level of concern about the consequences of falling is thought necessary to raise awareness and to encourage people towards participation in falls prevention programmes (Janz and Becker, 1984), there is growing consensus that high levels of concern about falls may be dysfunctional and possibly lead to avoidance of fall-related activities (Brouwer et al., 2004; Friedman et al., 2002; Howland et al., 1998; Legters, 2002; Murphy et al., 2002). The resulting reduction in activity may then result in physical deconditioning (concern about falls may be dysfunctional and possibly lead to avoidance of fall-related activities (Brouwer et al., 2004;

Delbaere *et al.*, 2004; Maki *et al.*, 1991; Myers *et al.*, 1996), poor quality of life (Arfken *et al.*, 1994; Lawrence *et al.*, 1998), social isolation (Arfken *et al.*, 1994; Howland *et al.*, 1998; Murphy *et al.*, 2002), depression and psychological distress (Arfken *et al.*, 1994; Chandler *et al.*, 1996; Howland *et al.*, 1998)).

Notes

1 www.sign.ac.uk/assets/sign142.pdf.
2 www.gov.uk/government/uploads/system/uploads/attachment_data/file/679885/ Structured_literature_review_report_falls_prevention.pdf.

References

Arfken CL, Lach HW, Birge SJ, Miller JP. (1994). The prevalence and correlates of fear of falling in elderly persons living in the community. *Am J Public Health*. 84(4): 565–70.

Auais M, French S, Alvarado B, Pirkle C, Belanger E, Guralnik J. (2017). Fear of falling predicts incidence of functional disability two years later: a perspective from an international cohort study. *J Gerontol A Biol Sci Med Sci*. December 6. doi:10.1093/gerona/glx237. [Epub ahead of print].

Auais M, Morin S, Nadeau L, Finch L, Mayo N. (2013). Changes in frailty-related characteristics of the hip fracture population and their implications for healthcare services: evidence from Quebec, Canada. *Osteoporos Int*. 24: 2713–24.

Austin N, Devine A, Dick I, Prince R, Bruce D. (2007). Fear of falling in older women: a longitudinal study of incidence, persistence and predictors. *J Am Geriatr Soc*. 55: 1598–603.

Bandura A. (1982). The assessment and predictive generality of self-percepts of efficacy. *J Behav Ther Exp Psychiatry*. 13(3): 195–9.

Barlow JH, Ellard DR, Hainsworth JM, Jones FR, Fisher A. (2005). A review of self-management interventions for panic disorders, phobias and obsessive-compulsive disorders. *Acta Psychiatr Scand*. 111(4): 272–85.

Beaupre LA, Binder EF, Cameron ID, Jones CA, Orwig D, Sherrington C, Magaziner J. (2013). Maximising functional recovery following hip fracture in frail seniors. *Best Pract Res Clin Rheumatol*. December; 27(6): 771–88. doi:10.1016/j.berh.2014.01.001.

Bentler SE, Liu L, Obrizan M, Cook EA, Wright KB, Geweke JF, Chrischilles EA, Pavlik CE, Wallace RB, Ohsfeldt RL, Jones MP, Rosenthal GE, Wolinsky FD. (2009). The aftermath of hip fracture: discharge placement, functional status change, and mortality. *Am J Epidemiol*. 170: 1290–9.

Bodenheimer T, Lorig K, Holman H, Grumbach K. (2002). Patient selfmanagement of chronic disease in primary care. *JAMA*. 288(19): 2469–75.

BonnerupVind A, Elkjaer Andersen H, Damgaard Pedersen K, Joergensen T, Schwarz P. (2010). The effect of a program of multifactorial fall prevention on health-related quality of life, functional ability, fear of falling and psychological well-being: a randomized controlled trial. *Aging Clin Exp Res*. 22: 249–54.

Boots AM, Maier AB, Stinissen P, Masson P, Lories RJ, De Keyser F. (2013). The influence of ageing on the development and management of rheumatoid arthritis. *Nat Rev Rheumatol*. October; 9(10): 604–13. doi:10.1038/nrrheum.2013.92. Epub 2013 June 18.

Brouwer B, Musselman K, Culham E. (2004). Physical function and health status among seniors with and without a fear of falling. *Gerontology*. 50(3): 135–41.

Chandler JM, Duncan PW, Sanders L, Studenski S. (1996). The fear of falling syndrome: relationship to falls, physical performance, and activities of daily living in frail older persons. *Topics in Geriatric Rehabilitation.* 11(3): 55–63.

Chang JT, Morton SC, Rubenstein LZ, Mojica WA, Maglione M, Suttorp MJ, Roth EA, Shekelle PG. (2004). Interventions for the prevention of falls in older adults: systematic review and meta-analysis of randomized controlled trials. *BMJ.* 328: 680–3.

Chen JS, Cameron ID, Simpson JM, Seibel MJ, March LM, Cumming RG, Lord SR, Sambrook PN. (2011). Low-trauma fractures indicate increased risk of hip fracture in frail older people. *J Bone Miner Res.* February; 26(2): 428–33. doi:10.1002/jbmr.216.

Choi JY, Cho KJ, Kim SW, Yoon SJ, Kang MG, Kim KI, Lee YK, Koo KH, Kim CH. (2017). Prediction of mortality and postoperative complications using the hip-multidimensional frailty score in elderly patients with hip fracture. *Sci Rep.* February 24; 7: 42966. doi:10.1038/srep42966.

Clancy A, Balteskard B, Perander B, Mahler M. (2015). Older persons' narrations on falls and falling: stories of courage and endurance. *Int J Qual Stud Health Well-being.* January 8; 10: 26123. doi:10.3402/qhw.v10.26123. eCollection 2015.

Clegg A, Young J, Iliffe S, Rikkert MO, Rockwood K. (2013). Frailty in elderly people. *Lancet.* 381(9868): 752–62. doi:10.1016/S0140-6736(12)62167-9.

Cooper C. (1992). Hip fractures in the elderly: a world-wide projection. *Osteoporosis International.* 2: 285–9.

Crow RS, Lohman MC, Pidgeon D, Bruce ML, Bartels SJ, Batsis JA. (2018). Frailty versus stopping elderly accidents, deaths and injuries initiative fall risk score: ability to predict future falls. *J Am Geriatr Soc.* February 10. doi:10.1111/jgs.15275. [Epub ahead of print].

Delbaere K, Crombez G, Vanderstraeten G, Willems T, Cambier D. (2004). Fear-related avoidance of activities, falls and physical frailty: a prospective community-based cohort study. *Age Ageing.* 33(4): 368–73.

Ensrud KE, Ewing SK, Fredman L, Hochberg MC, Cauley JA, Hillier TA, Cummings SR, Yaffe K, Cawthon PM; Study of Osteoporotic Fractures Research Group. (2010). Circulating 25-hydroxyvitamin D levels and frailty status in older women. *J Clin Endocrinol Metab.* December; 95(12): 5266–73. doi:10.1210/jc.2010-2317.

Fang X, Shi J, Song X, Mitnitski A, Tang Z, Wang C., Yu P, Rockwood K. (2012). Frailty in relation to the risk of falls, fractures, and mortality in older Chinese adults: results from the Beijing Longitudinal Study of Aging. *J Nutr Health Aging.* 16: 903–7. pmid: 23208030.

Freiberger E, Kemmler W, Siegrist M, Sieber C. (2016). Frailty and exercise interventions: evidence and barriers for exercise programs. *Z Gerontol Geriatr.* October; 49(7): 606–11. Epub 2016 September 21.

Freund T, Gensichen J, Goetz K, Szecsenyi J, Mahler C. (2013). Evaluating selfefficacy for managing chronic disease: psychometric properties of the six-item self-efficacy scale in Germany. *J Eval Clin Pract.* 19(1): 39–43.

Fried LP, Bandeen-Roche K, Chaves PH, Johnson BA. (2000). Preclinical mobility disability predicts incident mobility disability in older women. *The Journals of Gerontology. Series A, Biological Sciences and Medical Sciences.* 55: M43–M52.

Friedman SM, Munoz B, West SK, Rubin GS, Fried LP. (2002). Falls and fear of falling: which comes first? A longitudinal prediction model suggests strategies for primary and secondary prevention. *Journal of the American Geriatrics Society.* 50(8): 1329–35.

Gill TM, Allore HG, Hardy SE, Guo Z. (2006). The dynamic nature of mobility disability in older persons. *Journal of the American Geriatrics Society.* 54: 248–54.

Gillespie LD. (2004). Preventing falls in elderly people. *BMJ.* 328: 653–4.

Gillespie LD, Robertson MC, Gillespie WJ, Sherrington C, Gates S, Clemson LM, Lamb SE. (2012). Interventions for preventing falls in older people living in the community. *Cochrane Database Syst Rev.* 2012(9). doi:10.1002/14651858.CD007146.pub3.

Guccione AA. (1997). Osteoarthritis, comorbidity, and physical disability. In: Hamerman D (ed.), *Osteo-arthritis: public health implications for an aging population.* Baltimore, MD: The Johns Hopkins University Press, pp. 84–98.

Hadjistavropoulos T, Delbaere K, Fitzgerald TD. (2011). Reconceptualizing the role of fear of falling and balance confidence in fall risk. *J Aging Health.* 23(1): 3–23.

Halvarsson A, Olsson E, Farén E, Pettersson A, Ståhle A. (2011). Effects of new, individually adjusted, progressive balance group training for elderly people with fear of falling and tend to fall: a randomized controlled trial. *Clin Rehabil.* 25: 1021–31. doi:10.1177/v0269215511411937.

Hans D, Šteňová E, Lamy O. (2017). The Trabecular Bone Score (TBS) complements DXA and the FRAX as a fracture risk assessment tool in routine clinical practice. *Curr Osteoporos Rep.* December; 15(6): 521–31. doi:10.1007/s11914-017-0410-z.

Healey F, Monro A, Cockram A, Adams V, Heseltine D. (2004). Using targeted risk factor reduction to prevent falls in older in-patients: a randomised controlled trial. *Age Ageing.* 33: 1–5.

Healey F, Scobie S, Oliver D, Pryce A, Thomson R, Glampson B. (2008). Falls in English and Welsh hospitals: a national observational study based on retrospective analysis of 12 months of patient safety incident reports. *Qual Saf Health Care.* 17: 424–30.

Howland J, Lachman M, Peterson E, Cote J, Kasten L, Jette A. (1998). Covariates of fear of falling and associated activity curtailment. *Gerontologist.* 38: 549–55.

Janz NK, Becker MH. (1984). The health belief model: a decade later. *Health Education Quarterly.* 11(1): 1–47.

Jellesmark A, Herling SF, Egerod I, Beyer N. (2012). Fear of falling and changed functional ability following hip fracture among community-dwelling elderly people: an explanatory sequential mixed method study. *Disabil Rehabil.* 34(25): 2124–31. doi:10.3109/0963828 8.2012.673685. Epub 2012 April 26.

Kanis JA; on behalf of World Health Organization Scientific Group. (2007). *Assessment of osteoporosis at the primary health care level.* WHO Scientific Group Technical report. World Health Organization Collaborating Centre for Metabolic Bone Diseases, University of Sheffield, Sheffield, UK. www.sheffield.ac.uk/FRAX/pdfs/WHO_Technical_Report.pdf (accessed 17 May 2018).

Kannus P, Sievanen H, Palvanen M, Jarvinen T, Parkkari J. (2005). Prevention of falls and consequent injuries in elderly people. *Lancet.* 366: 1885–93.

Kendrick D, Kumar A, Carpenter H, Zijlstra G, Skelton DA, Cook JR *et al.* (2014). Exercise for reducing fear of falling in older people living in the community. *The Cochrane Database of Systematic Reviews.* 11. doi:10.1002/14651858.CD009848.pub2.

Krishnan M, Beck S, Havelock W, Eeles E, Hubbard RE, Johansen A. (2014). Predicting outcome after hip fracture: using a frailty index to integrate comprehensive geriatric assessment results. *Age Ageing.* January; 43(1): 122–6. doi:10.1093/ageing/aft084. Epub 2013 July 5.

Lawrence RH, Tennstedt SL, Kasten LE, Shih J, Howland J, Jette AM. (1998). Intensity and correlates of fear of falling and hurting oneself in the next year: baseline findings from a Roybal center fear of falling intervention. *Journal of Aging and Health.* 10(3): 267–86.

Lee F, Mackenzie L, James C. (2008). Perceptions of older people living in the community about their fear of falling. *Disabil Rehabil.* 30: 1803–11.

Legters, K. (2002). Fear of falling. *Physical Therapy.* 82(3): 264–72.

Li G, Papaioannou A, Thabane L, Cheng J, Adachi JD. (2016). frailty change and major osteoporotic fracture in the elderly: data from the Global Longitudinal Study of Osteoporosis in Women 3-Year Hamilton Cohort. *J Bone Miner Res.* April; 31(4): 718–24. doi:10.1002/jbmr.2739. Epub 2015 November 30.

Maki BE, Holliday PJ, Topper AK. (1991). Fear of falling and postural performance in the elderly. *Journals of Gerontology.* 46(4): M123–M131.

Malini FM, Lourenço RA, Lopes CS. (2016). Prevalence of fear of falling in older adults, and its associations with clinical, functional and psychosocial factors: the Frailty in Brazilian Older People – Rio de Janeiro Study. *Geriatr Gerontol Int.* March; 16(3): 336–44. doi:10.1111/ggi.12477. Epub 2015 April 14.

Michelon E, Blaum C, Semba RD, Xue Q-L, Ricks MO, Fried LP. (2006). Vitamin and carotenoid status in older women: associations with the frailty syndrome. *J Gerontol A Biol Sci Med Sci.* 61A: 600–7.

Misra D, Felson DT, Silliman RA, Nevitt M, Lewis CE, Torner J, Neogi T. (2015). Knee osteoarthritis and frailty: findings from the Multicenter Osteoarthritis Study and Osteoarthritis Initiative. *J Gerontol A Biol Sci Med Sci.* March; 70(3): 339–44. doi:10.1093/gerona/glu102. Epub 2014 July 25.

Murphy J, Isaacs B. (1982). The post-fall syndrome: a study of 36 elderly patients. *Gerontology.* 28: 265–70.

Murphy SL, Dubin JA, Gill TM. (2003). The development of fear of falling among community-living older women: predisposing factors and subsequent fall events. *The Journals of Gerontology Series A: Biological Sciences and Medical Sciences.* 58(10): M943–M947.

Murphy SL, Williams CS, Gill TM. (2002). Characteristics associated with fear of falling and activity restriction in community-living older persons. *J Am Geriatr Soc.* 50(3): 516–20.

Myers AM, Powell LE, Maki BE, Holliday PJ, Brawley LR, Sherk W. (1996). Psychological indicators of balance confidence: relationship to actual and perceived abilities. *Journals of Gerontology Series A Biological Sciences and Medical Sciences.* 51(1): M37–M43.

NIH Consensus Development Panel on Osteoporosis Prevention, Diagnosis, and Therapy. (2001). Osteoporosis prevention, diagnosis, and therapy. *JAMA.* 285: 785–95.

Nowak A, Hubbard RE. (2009). Falls and frailty: lessons from complex systems. *R Soc Med.* March; 102(3): 98–102. doi:10.1258/jrsm.2009.080274.

Park-Lee E, Fredman L, Hochberg M, Faulkner K. (2009). Positive affect and incidence of frailty in elderly women caregivers and noncaregivers: results of Caregiver-Study of Osteoporotic Fractures. *J Am Geriatr Soc.* April; 57(4): 627–33. doi:10.1111/j.1532-5415.2009.02183.x.

Parry SW, Bamford C, Deary V, Finch TL, Gray J, MacDonald C, McMeekin P, Sabin NJ, Steen IN, Whitney SL, McColl EM. (2016). Cognitive-behavioural therapy-based intervention to reduce fear of falling in older people: therapy development and randomised controlled trial – the Strategies for Increasing Independence, Confidence and Energy (STRIDE) study. *Health Technol Assess.* July; 20(56): 1–206. doi:10.3310/hta20560.

Patil R, Uusi-Rasi K, Kannus P, Karinkanta S, Sievänen H. (2014). Concern about falling in older women with a history of falls: associations with health, functional ability, physical activity and quality of life. *Gerontology.* 60(1): 22–30. doi:10.1159/000354335. Epub 2013 October 8.

Puts MT, Visser M, Twisk JW, Deeg DJH, Lips P. (2005). Endocrine and inflammatory markers as predictors of frailty. *Clin Endocrinol* (Oxford). 63: 403–11.

Rizzoli R, Branco J, Brandi ML, Boonen S, Bruyere O, Cacoub P, Cooper C, Diez-Perez A, Duder J, Fielding RA, Harvey NC, Hiligsmann M, Kanis JA, Petermans J, Ringe JD, Tsouderos Y, Weinman J, Reginster JY. (2014). Management of osteoporosis in the oldest old. *Osteoporosis International.* 25: 2507–29.

Rochat S, Büla CJ, Martin E, Seematter-Bagnoud L, Karmaniola A, Aminian K, Piot-Ziegler C, Santos-Eggimann B. (2010). What is the relationship between fear of falling and gait in well-functioning older persons aged 65 to 70 years? *Arch Phys Med Rehabil.* 91(6): 879–84.

Royal College of Physicians. (2017). Falls and fragility fracture audit programme (FFAP). National audit of inpatient falls: audit report 2017, November, www.rcplondon.ac.uk/projects/outputs/naif-audit-report-2017.

Runge M. (1998). *Gehstörungen, Stürze, Hüftfrakturen.* Berlin, Heidelberg: Springer-Verlag, Schulz, K. F.

Scheffer AC, Schuurmans MJ, van Dijk N, van der Hooft T, de Rooij SE. (2008). Fear of falling: measurement strategy, prevalence, risk factors and consequences among older persons. *Age and Ageing.* 37: 19–24.

Schwartz AV, Nevitt MC, Brown BW Jr, Kelsey JL. (2005). Increased falling as a risk factor for fracture among older women: the study of osteoporotic fractures. *Am J Epidemiol.* January 15; 161(2): 180–5.

Seematter-Bagnoud L, Santos-Eggimann B, Rochat S, Martin E, Karmaniola A, Aminian K, Piot-Ziegler C, Büla CJ. (2010). Vulnerability in high-functioning persons aged 65 to 70 years: the importance of the fear factor. *Aging Clin Exp Res.* June; 22(3): 212–18. doi:10.3275/6705. Epub 2009 November 27.

Simmons LA, Wolever RQ. (2013). Integrative health coaching and motivational interviewing: synergistic approaches to behavior change in healthcare. *Glob Adv Health Med.* July; 2(4): 28–35. doi:10.7453/gahmj.2013.037.

Szulc P, Bouxsein ML; International Osteoporosis Foundation. (2010). *Vertebral Fracture Initiative. Part I. Overview of osteoporosis: Epidemiology and clinical management.* www.iof-bonehealth.org/sites/default/files/PDFs/Vertebral%20Fracture%20Initiative/IOF_VFI-Part_I-Manuscript.pdf.

Tinetti ME, Powell L. (1993). Fear of falling and low self-efficacy: a case of dependence in elderly persons. *J Gerontol.* 48 (Spec. No.): 35–38.

Tom SE, Adachi JD, Anderson FA Jr, Boonen S, Chapurlat RD, Compston JE, Cooper C, Gehlbach SH, Greenspan SL, Hooven FH, Nieves JW, Pfeilschifter J, Roux C, Silverman S, Wyman A, LaCroix AZ; GLOW Investigators. (2013). Frailty and fracture, disability, and falls: a multiple country study from the global longitudinal study of osteoporosis in women. *J Am Geriatr Soc.* March; 61(3): 327–34. doi:10.1111/jgs.12146. Epub 2013 January 25.

Wei F, Hester AL. (2014). Gender difference in falls among adults treated in emergency departments and outpatient clinics. *J Gerontol Geriatr Res.* 3: 152.

Williams C. (2002). A cognitive–behavioural therapy assessment model for use in everyday clinical practice. *Adv Psychiatr Treat.* 8: 172–9. doi:10.1192/apt.8.3.172.

Writing Group for the ISCD Position Development Conference. (2004). Position statement: executive summary. The Writing Group for the International Society for Clinical Densitometry (ISCD) Position Development Conference. *J. Clin. Densitom.* 7: 7–12.

Youde J, Husk J, Lowe D, Grant R, Potter J, Martin F. (2009). The national clinical audit of falls and bone health: the clinical management of hip fracture patients. *Injury.* November; 40(11): 1226–30. doi:10.1016/j.injury.2009.06.167. Epub 2009 July 31.

Zidén L, Häggblom-Kronlöf G, Gustafsson S, Lundin-Olsson L, Dahlin-Ivanoff S. (2014). Physical function and fear of falling 2 years after the health-promoting randomized controlled trial: elderly persons in the risk zone. *Gerontologist.* June; 54(3): 387–97. doi:10.1093/GERONT/GNT078. Epub 2013 August 1.

Zijlstra G. (2007). Interventions to reduce fear of falling in community-living older people: a systematic review. *J Am Geriatr Soc.* 55: 603–15.

Zijlstra GA, Van Haastregt JCM, Van Rossum E, Van Eijk JTM, Yardley L, Kempen GIJM. (2007). Interventions to reduce fear of falling in community-living older people: a systematic review. *J Am Geriatr Soc.* 55: 603–15.

Zunzunegui MV, Alvarado BE, Guerra R, Gómez JF, Ylli A, Guralnik JM; Imias Research Group. (2015). The mobility gap between older men and women: the embodiment of gender. *Arch Gerontol Geriatr.* September–October; 61(2): 140–8. doi:10.1016/j. archger.2015.06.005. Epub 2015 June 17.

4

SURGICAL OUTCOMES, COGNITIVE FRAILTY AND DELIRIUM

Aim

Tipping someone with cognitive impairment and frailty into delirium is a good example where an effort to maximise somebody's assets and resilience might help prevent negative outcomes. A shock which healthy adults can cope with, such as infection or surgery, can be catastrophic for certain individuals. This chapter reviews the current evidence for surgical outcomes and delirium for people who are frail.

Introduction

Geriatric syndromes are important prognostic factors for postoperative complications. A recent study, involving review of 44 prospective studies reporting prognostic factors associated with postoperative complications (composite outcome of medical and surgical complications), functional decline, mortality, post-hospitalisation discharge destination, and prolonged hospitalisation among older adults undergoing elective surgery identified potentially modifiable prognostic factors (e.g. frailty, depressive symptoms and smoking) associated with developing postoperative complications that can be targeted preoperatively to optimise care (Watt *et al.*, 2018). As I introduced right at the beginning of this book, frailty reflects the life-long accumulation of deficits, thus defining the greater or lesser state of vulnerability of the individual. This Rockwood and Mitnitski contribution is seminal.

Such (more or less overt) accentuated susceptibility to stressors represents the biological background where delirium might find its onset (Bellelli *et al.*, 2017). For example, an infection, a background of frailty and dementia, and a hospital admission could easily tip someone over the finishing line for becoming delirious. In the absence of targeted interventions, the progression of frailty is marked by increased risk of adverse health-related outcomes (Fougère *et al.*, 2017). A clear illustration of this is the emergence of delirium in a patient undergoing a surgical operation. It is important that we can identify those people who are frail early and give them the right care in hospital to ensure that they live well with frailty and avoid any of the known risks. This matters because admission to hospital can be disruptive, and can bring its own problems for someone who is showing features of frailty.

Surgical outcomes

Despite a growing literature that demonstrates strong independent associations between frailty and adverse outcomes, few interventions have been tested to improve the outcomes of frail surgical patients, and most available studies are at substantial risk of bias. McIsaac and colleagues (2017) have argued that 'multi-center, low risk of bias, studies of perioperative exercise are needed, while substantial efforts are required to develop and test other interventions to improve the outcomes of frail people having surgery'. Given the fact that the elderly population in many jurisdictions continues to grow exponentially, it is of utmost importance for frailty assessments to be implemented into clinical practice in order to predict clinical outcomes and to intervene appropriately with inpatient care. A consensus must be made to eliminate variations in definitions of frailty in order to create a universal tool able to assess the status of patients during surgical consults, admissions and peri/postoperative care (Stoicea *et al.*, 2016). Novel interdisciplinary rehabilitation programmes need to be developed together with geriatricians, neurologists, dieticians and other specialists in the comorbidities that are frequently met in frail patients (Gielen and Simm, 2017).

Lack of knowledge about frailty is a key barrier in the use of frailty assessments and the majority of respondents agreed that they would benefit from further training (Eamer *et al.*, 2017). (I introduced a notion of 'frailty awareness' back in Chapter 1.) Elderly patients frequently present with surgical emergencies to healthcare providers, and outcomes in this group of patients remain poor. Contributing factors include frailty, pre-existing comorbidity, polypharmacy, delayed diagnosis, and lack of timely and consultant-led treatment (Torrance *et al.*, 2015). A risk stratification approach for these patients serves a number of functions. Not all elderly patients have a frailty phenotype, which suggests that frailty is not an inevitable consequence of ageing and as such, may be amenable to treatment (Oakland *et al.*, 2016). The presence of a frailty phenotype has potential significance in an elderly surgical population as peri-operative frailty related interventions may improve outcomes.

Torrance *et al.* (2015, p. 55) describe:

> Identification of patients in whom treatment would be futile or associated with high risk is needed to avoid unnecessary interventions and to give patients and carers realistic expectations. The use of multidisciplinary teams to identify common postoperative complications and age-specific syndromes

is paramount. Prevention of complications is preferable to rescue treatment due to the high proportion of patients who fail to recover from adverse events. Even with successful surgical treatment, long-term functional decline and increased dependency are common. More research into emergency surgery in the elderly is needed to improve care for this growing group of vulnerable patients.

Often surgeons assess patients as surgical candidates by an 'eyeball test' that is subjective and does not truly correlate with the risk of postoperative complications (Hii *et al.*, 2015). Indeed, physicians' conceptualisation of frailty as dynamic and on a spectrum, picking up on a 'clinical gestalt' of frailty, introduces more flexibility into frailty assessment than existing objective tools can provide (Korenvain *et al.*, 2018). Measuring frailty before surgery in older adults may confer added risk stratification beyond age and traditional perioperative risk factors. It is therefore increasingly important to use validated measures to appraise frailty preoperatively where potential exists to modify treatment options and adjust expectations for recovery before surgery (Cooper *et al.*, 2016).

Frail people can undergo surgical procedures as frequently as those without frailty, but recent findings suggest that being frail can be independently associated with an increased length of hospital stay and a higher chance of death, than someone less frail (Hewitt *et al.*, 2015). In elective general surgery, frailty has been associated with an increase in postoperative complications (Dasgupta *et al.*, 2009; Revenig *et al.*, 2013; Robinson *et al.*, 2009), and an increased use of social care following discharge from hospital (Robinson *et al.*, 2011; Makary *et al.*, 2010).

Within the older surgical population, the process of preoperative assessment provides an opportunity for proactive recognition of the frailty syndrome. The preoperative assessment process can be considered to serve two broad purposes: first, to risk stratify patients in order that health professionals, patients and their relatives or care partners are fully informed of the inherent risks in undergoing a procedure; second, in order that modifiable factors are proactively identified and optimised preoperatively, thus improving the patient's likelihood of a successful outcome (Partridge *et al.*, 2012).

Surgical outcomes in specific scenarios

It is interesting to look at surgical outcomes in specific scenarios, and I can only sample here a very small sample of current published examples.

Gastric cancer is the fourth most common malignancy and the second most common cause of cancer-related deaths worldwide. As the ageing population expands, older patients are increasingly presenting for gastric cancer surgery. Frailty, as a predictor for an adverse outcome after surgery, has gained attention in recent years. However, few studies have used frailty to predict postoperative complications and the prognoses of elderly patients with gastric cancer (Lu *et al.*, 2017).

Sarcopenia or muscle mass loss is a component of frailty which seems to be accelerated when diabetes is present (Abdelhafiz *et al.*, 2016). Recently, sarcopenia has been associated with poor outcomes in urological patients; however, it requires imaging studies to determine the loss of muscle mass (Psutka *et al.*, 2014). Urologists could use sarcopenia in addition to frailty index when imaging studies are available, and loss of muscle mass can be determined to supplement the frailty index. Whatever frailty index urologists choose to implement in clinical settings, it is important for them to be cognisant of the fact that frailty is associated with significantly increased risk of adverse surgical outcomes (Isharwal *et al.*, 2017). Most clinicians are easily convinced that presurgical interventions focused on sarcopenic and malnourished patients are good for patient care, making developing programmes that are financially viable 'a must' (Friedman *et al.*, 2015).

Hip fracture is significantly associated with functional deterioration, early nursing home admission and premature death (Stevens, 2005). Surgical fixation has been associated with a reduced length of hospital stay, improved rehabilitation, better pain control and fracture healing without leg shortening in older adults admitted for a hip fracture (Handoll *et al.*, 2008).

Cognitive frailty

It is important to realise that there can be significant barriers to communication which may include where someone has additional care, support or communication needs such as a cognitive impairment, for example dementia.

Cognitive frailty was a notion proposed by Panza and colleagues (2006) when these authors examined the risks of decreased cognitive functions modulated by vascular factors. Subsequent studies revealed that physical factors and cognition are crucial elements in predicting risk of death (Panza *et al.*, 2006, 2011; Pilotto *et al.*, 2012). Cognitive frailty, as a concept, faces some challenges, mainly because the causal relationship between physical frailty and cognitive impairment over time is not yet fully understood (Montero-Odasso *et al.*, 2016). Although the emergence of cognitive frailty reflects a verifiable improvement in preventing a poor prognosis of ageing, many experts in the field have provided beneficial suggestions for clarifying the definition of cognitive frailty (Buchman and Bennett, 2013; Dartigues and Amieva, 2014).

The identification of 'cognitive frailty' raises the possibility that different groups of patients may have markedly different outcomes (see Figure 4.1).

To differentiate cognitive impairment from dementia in the absence of physical frailty, a consensus on the definition of cognitive frailty was reached by the International Academy on Nutrition and Aging and the International Association of Gerontology and Geriatrics in April, 2013 (Kelaiditi *et al.*, 2013).

In 2001, the term 'cognitive frailty' had been incidentally used by Paganini-Hill and colleagues examining 'clock-drawing test' performance and its association with several protective and risk factors for Alzheimer's disease in an older cohort (Paganini-Hill *et al.*, 2001). In 2006, this clinical label was first used to indicate a particular state of cognitive vulnerability in mild cognitive impairment and other similar clinical entities exposed to the risk modulated by vascular factors with a

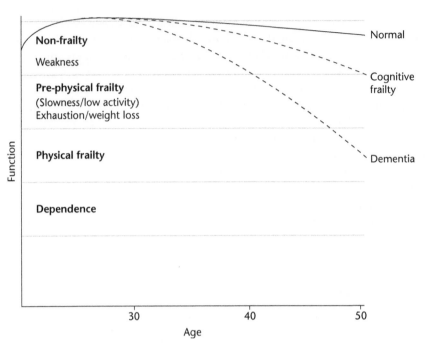

FIGURE 4.1 The components of cognitive frailty and different trajectories of both physical and cognitive functions under specific conditions

Source: redrawn from Figure 1, p. 3 of Ruan Q, Yu Z, Chen M, Bao Z, Li J, He W. (2015). Cognitive frailty, a novel target for the prevention of elderly dependency. *Ageing Res Rev*. March; 20: 1–10. doi:10.1016/j.arr.2014.12.004. Epub 2014 December 30.

subsequent increased progression to dementia, particularly vascular dementia (Panza *et al.*, 2006). It might be that individuals who are cognitively frail have the highest risks of IADL (instrumental activities of daily living) limitations (see Table 4.1). Future investigation is necessary to determine whether this population is at increased risk for incidence of disability or mortality.

The overall concept of examining the specific cognitive correlates of frailty is interesting, and may indeed shed light on a more comprehensive model of frailty that details a specific neuropsychological profile (Amanzio *et al.*, 2017). Evidence derives from data supporting the existence of shared risk factors. For example, brain infarcts and high pro-inflammatory cytokines such as tumour necrosis factor-α, interleukin-6 and C-reactive protein are associated with both impaired cognition and frailty syndrome. In a longitudinal study of 104 cognitively intact participants, Silbert and colleagues found an association between progression of white matter hyper-intensity on brain magnetic resonance imaging and a decline in gait and cognitive function over 13 years of follow-up (Silbert *et al.*, 2008). These data perhaps suggest that inflammation, brain infarcts and other pathological factors might be contributing to both the development of frailty and the onset of cognitive decline in older adults.

TABLE 4.1 Comparisons with IADL limitations and confounding factors between the participants who were robust, or had physical frailty, or cognitive frailty with mean (SD) or number (percentage)

	Robust	Physical frailty	Cognitive frailty
IADL items			
IADL decline, yes	1,935 (25.3)	203 (32.0)	53 (48.6)
Using a bus or a train, no	585 (7.6)	83 (13.1)	25 (22.9)
Grocery shopping, no	286 (3.7)	49 (7.7)	20 (18.3)
Management of finances, no	704 (9.2)	60 (9.5)	25 (22.9)
Demographic variables			
Age, years	72.9 (5.2)	78.2 (5.8)	77.6 (6.1)
Sex, male	3,719 (48.5)	267 (42.1)	44 (40.4)
Education, years	11.9 (2.5)	11.0 (2.7)	10.3 (2.4)
Chronic medical conditions			
Hypertension, yes	3,390 (44.3)	342 (53.9)	50 (45.9)
Heart disease, yes	1,231 (16.1)	167 (26.3)	26 (23.9)
Osteoarthritis, yes	1,280 (16.7)	180 (28.4)	18 (16.5)
Diabetes, yes	903 (11.8)	136 (21.5)	24 (22.0)
Medications, number	2.4 (2.4)	4.1 (3.3)	3.9 (3.0)
Hospitalisation during 3 months, yes	108 (1.4)	21 (3.3)	10 (9.2)
Life-styles			
Hobby and/or sports activity, no	1,400 (18.3)	287 (45.3)	57 (52.3)
Alcohol use, no	4,135 (54.0)	421 (66.4)	79 (72.5)
Psychosocial factors			
Geriatric Depression Scale-15, score	2.5 (2.4)	4.8 (3.2)	5.0 (3.2)
Live alone, yes	878 (11.5)	105 (16.6)	18 (16.5)

Source: adapted from Shimada *et al.*, 2016, p. 733, Table 2.

Some evidence indicates that the underlying neuropathological mechanisms associated with Alzheimer's disease begin a decade or more before the emergence of cognitive impairment (Sperling *et al.*, 2011). This understanding has had a substantial impact on the conduct of clinical trials related to Alzheimer's disease, since it is hypothesised that disease-modifying therapies are likely to be more successful when administered early in the course of disease. Findings raise the possibility that frailty and Alzheimer's disease may share common aetiologies.

The ageing brain is also characterised by structural and functional changes to microglial cells, which are the resident immune cell population of the CNS (central nervous system) and are the CNS equivalent of macrophages. They are activated by brain injury and local and systemic inflammation and become primed (hyper-responsive) to small stimuli with ageing, which can potentially cause damage and neuronal death (Luo *et al.*, 2010; Streit, 2006; Cunningham *et al.*, 2005). This is not only a limitation of brain frailty, but also that of other organs and systems, since the two most recognised models of frailty, the phenotypic model of Fried or the cumulative deficit model, use general functional indicators, as in the former, or an aggregate of deficits in clinical and laboratory parameters where only some assimilate to central nervous system functions, as in the latter (Cano, 2015).

Accumulating evidence from observational studies supports a *temporal association* between frailty, cognitive impairment and dementia. In a prospective cohort study of elderly people without cognitive impairment at baseline, the investigators reported that frailty was associated with an increased risk of the development of mild cognitive impairment during 12 years of follow-up (Boyle *et al.*, 2010). Together with prior studies showing an association between frailty, clinical Alzheimer's disease (AD), and AD pathology, these data may suggest that physical frailty and cognitive impairment share a common underlying pathogenesis (Boyle *et al.*, 2010). Emerging literature indicates that delirium is a strong predictor of new-onset dementia as well as acceleration of existing cognitive decline. This is consistent across different settings: after hospitalisation; in those with dementia; in postoperative patients; after critical care; and in community populations (Richardson *et al.*, 2017).

Currently optimal treatment to prevent or delay cognitive decline, mild cognitive impairment (MCI) or dementia is uncertain. Fink and colleagues (2018) reviewed current evidence on the efficacy and harms of pharmacologic interventions to prevent or delay cognitive decline, MCI or dementia in adults with normal cognition or MCI. The authors concluded that current evidence does not support use of the studied pharmacologic treatments for cognitive protection in persons with normal cognition or MCI. While pre-existing frailty and cause of delirium are not readily modifiable risk factors, poor recognition by treating physicians early in the course of delirium may be, suggesting that a potential remedy for the poor outcomes associated with delirium may be within the grasp of attentive practitioners (Andrew *et al.*, 2005). Compared to robust non-cognitively impaired individuals, physical pre-frailty with cognitive impairment was associated with a two-fold increased prevalence and incidence of functional disability, a two-fold increased incidence of poor QOL, and 1.8-fold increased mortality risks (Feng *et al.*, 2017). The Hispanic Established Populations for the Epidemiologic Study of the Elderly, involving five south-western U.S. states, demonstrated that frailty and cognitive impairment affect mortality differently when they occur independently compared with when they are present together (Cano *et al.*, 2012).

Hypoglycaemia, frailty and dementia have a reciprocal relationship which may lead to a viscious circle (see Figure 4.2). Hypoglycaemic events seem to be common in older people with diabetes, especially in those who are frail and suffered from significant weight loss. This group of patients currently appear to be over-treated and seem to be inappropriately using medications that likely increase the risk of hypoglycaemia.

Resilience and 'cognitive reserve'

The cellular mechanisms underlying resilience, in relation to cognitive frailty and reserve, are actually quite fascinating. There is converging evidence that degenerative

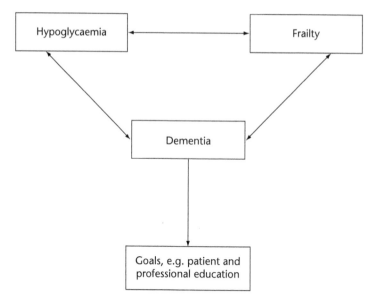

FIGURE 4.2 Interaction of hypoglycaemia, frailty and dementia comprising a vicious circle and considerations for clinical implications

Source: redrawn from Figure 1, p. 1533 of Abdelhafiz AH, McNicholas E, Sinclair AJ. (2016). Hypoglycemia, frailty and dementia in older people with diabetes: reciprocal relations and clinical implications. *J Diabetes Complications.* November–December; 30(8): 1548–54. doi:10.1016/j.jdiacomp. 2016.07.027. Epub 2016 July 27.

processes of the entorhinal–hippocampal formation occur at very early stages of Alzheimer's disease (Braak and Braak, 1991, 1997). Atrophy of the medial temporal lobe, particularly the parahippocampal and hippocampal regions, seems associated with memory loss (Laakso *et al.*, 2000; Pennanen *et al.*, 2004). Thus, reduction in hippocampal volume represents one of the structural hallmarks of incipient AD (Chetelat and Baron, 2003; Kantarci and Jack, 2003; Wolf *et al.*, 2004). From a clinical standpoint, the amnestic type of mild cognitive impairment (Petersen *et al.*, 1999, 2001) is at present the most valid concept indicative of incipient or early AD (Morris *et al.*, 2001; Grundman *et al.*, 2003; Crocco and Loewenstein, 2005).

Risk reduction action appears to be important in cognitive frailty, as it so clearly is for dementia. A parallel area of research is whether resilience occurs in cognitive neurology due to a 'cognitive reserve'. Reserve refers to the phenomenon of relatively preserved cognition in disproportion to the extent of neuropathology, e.g. in Alzheimer's disease. A putative functional neural substrate underlying reserve is global functional connectivity of the left lateral frontal cortex (Franzmeier *et al.*, 2017). The beneficial effects of education, IQ and other cognitive reserve promoting factors had been found to be most pronounced in preclinical and prodromal stages of AD (i.e. MCI), indicating that the ability to better cope with brain pathology might be highest earlier in the disease course (Scarmeas *et al.*, 2004; Stern, 2002).

Delirium and frailty

Delirium is characterised by fluctuating disturbances of consciousness, disorientation and perception abnormalities, alongside impaired thinking and speech, that typically settles after several days (e.g. Inouye, 2006; Saczynski *et al.*, 2012). Frailty and delirium share several commonalities but also have specific differences. Both should be considered as multifactorial health conditions, characterised by multiple risk factors and causation which are not necessarily specific to a given organ system failure (Bellelli *et al.*, 2017). Cognitive impairment is the decline of intellectual function and can be acute onset (delirium), chronic (dementia) or acute on chronic. Delirium is a concept all surgeons will be familiar with, especially in elective orthopaedic or cardiothoracic surgery, where, in the latter, it is estimated to develop in up to 75 per cent of patients postoperatively (Moug *et al.*, 2016). However, delirium remains a clinical diagnosis which is often unrecognised and easily overlooked despite recent impressive awareness campaigns. Recognition of the disorder necessitates brief cognitive screening and astute clinical observation. Key diagnostic features include an acute onset and fluctuating course of symptoms, inattention, impaired consciousness and disturbance of cognition (e.g. disorientation, memory impairment, language changes) (Inouye *et al.*, 2014).

Delirium is statistically associated with frailty: people with frailty and delirium are at a higher risk of death than delirious patients who are not frail (Eeles *et al.*, 2012). Recognition of prevalent delirium at initial patient assessment may be difficult owing to lack of available informant or because the fluctuating nature of the condition means that a period of observation is required: establishing the time course of behavioural change is a key component of validated screening tools such as the Confusion Assessment Method and the 4AT (Pendlebury *et al.*, 2017). Risk factors for delirium that have so far been identified include: increased age, sensory deprivation (visual or hearing impairment), sleep deprivation, social isolation, physical restraint, use of bladder catheter, iatrogenic adverse events, polypharmacy (more than three new medications added), use of psychoactive drugs, comorbidities, severe illness (especially infection, fracture or stroke), prior cognitive impairment, temperature abnormality (fever or hypothermia), dehydration, malnutrition and low serum albumin (review, Siddiqi *et al.*, 2016). Despite successful reductions in incident delirium by about a third, anticipated reductions in mortality or admissions to long-term care have not been conclusively observed (Teale and Young, 2015). Frailty is also increasingly recognised as an important prognostic factor in patients with chronic diseases (Abdullah *et al.*, 2017). Consequently, it has been demonstrated that frailty is associated with a significantly increased likelihood of postoperative mortality and morbidity (Velanovich *et al.*, 2013).

Frailty and delirium, though seemingly distinct syndromes, both result in significant negative health outcomes in older patients. Frailty and delirium may be different clinical expressions of a shared vulnerability to stress in older patients and future research will determine whether this vulnerability is age-related, pathological, genetic or environmental or, most likely, a combination of all of these factors (Quinlan *et al.*, 2011). Death and institutionalisation as endpoints may, therefore, represent non-modifiable manifestations of frailty, and be relatively insensitive to a reduction in incident delirium, although a recent study has questioned the association of delirium with frailty (Joosten *et al.*, 2014). A possible relationship between the two syndromes is also supported by the higher prevalence of frailty amongst individuals with delirium (Verloo *et al.*, 2016), and reports that frailty is associated with poorer functional outcomes and increased mortality in delirium (Eeles *et al.*, 2012).

If prior pathology/loss of innervation contributes more significantly to delirium susceptibility than '**inflammatory priming**', this predicts that patients and animals with prior pathology would also show increased susceptibility to insults that are not inflammatory in nature and this is certainly the case with delirium: old age, cognitive impairment and frailty predispose to all causes of delirium (MacLullich and Hall, 2011; Fong *et al.*, 2009). Recent findings have suggested that the progressive loss of pre-synaptic terminals and the accumulation of white matter pathology shown here represent significant brain disconnectivity and quantifiable loss of 'brain reserve' (Satz, 1993). Synaptic loss is a strong correlate of cognitive decline and neuronal pathology occurs many years before cognitive impairment in AD (Terry, 2000).

Post-operative cognitive decline (POCD)

Post-operative cognitive dysfunction (POCD) is a condition characterised by a decline in memory and other cognitive functions following surgery and anaesthesia. First described in patients undergoing cardiac surgery (Folks *et al.*, 1988; Shaw *et al.*, 1987) and later major non-cardiac surgery (Moller *et al.*, 1998), POCD is a subtle condition reliably diagnosed only by neuropsychological testing and describes cognitive deficits that can be permanent. POCD is known to occur in all age groups and after any invasive surgery, with minor procedures being adequate to initiate neuroinflammation in older subjects (Rosczyk *et al.*, 2008). Traditional preoperative evaluation strategies risk-stratify patients based on compromise in single organ systems. Although single organ evaluation cannot be ignored in the aged patient, recognition of preoperative markers depicting the unique vulnerability of the geriatric patient (e.g. frailty, disability and comorbidity) may provide additional insight in predicting poor outcomes; thus aiding preoperative decision making (Robinson *et al.*, 2009). The constellation of frailty, disability and comorbidity are widely recognised to predict poor outcomes in elderly hospitalised patients.

Prehabilitation

The development of delirium is undoubtedly a complex process resulting from the interplay of various individual and environmental risk factors together with individual vulnerability (Ford, 2016). Work has previously identified independent factors thought to precipitate delirium in vulnerable adults (Inouye and Charpentier, 1996). Delirium is an important frailty syndrome, so it is important that it can be prevented. Understanding the nature of frailty may facilitate our understanding of long-term outcomes after intensive care, as well as being a trigger for considering the prognostic implications and the need to consider discussions with patients and their care partners and how the patient's own goals and expectations of care could be established around this information (Athari *et al.*, 2017). Specifically, there is initial evidence that **prehabilitation** may be used to reduce morbidity and mortality in frail patients. Notably, Harari and colleagues found that the introduction of a comprehensive geriatric assessment service resulted in a clinically significant decrease in medical complications and hospital length of stay (Harari *et al.*, 2007). However, at present, most recent guidelines are unable to conclusively support the use of prehabilitation as standard practice (Griffiths *et al.*, 2014).

The development of delirium is undoubtedly a complex process resulting from the interplay of various individual and environmental risk factors together with individual vulnerability (Ford, 2016). Delirium is common. As many as 20 to 50 per cent of the patients in an intensive care unit (ICU) without mechanical ventilation will have at least one episode of delirium during their stay. If a patient is receiving mechanical ventilation, the rate is as high as 80 per cent. In the neuro-critical care setting, the occurrence of delirium is also quite common, with rates of 19 to 70 per cent reported (Haymore and Patel, 2016). Although a single event can precipitate delirium, it is more common for multiple factors to interact and a multifactorial model of delirium has been established to help illustrate how delirium is precipitated in people at risk (Inouye and Charpentier, 1996).

The importance of using assets to build up resilience through 'prehabilitation' cannot be underestimated here. This can be viewed as altering the state of the **'frailty fulcrum'** introduced in Chapter 1. The importance of adequate nutritional support (Doig *et al.*, 2008), the value of sedation interruption (Schweickert *et al.*, 2009) coupled with early mobilisation (Kress, 2009) and physiotherapy (Salisbury *et al.*, 2010) to prevent physical deconditioning, and the psychological consequences of critical illness for both patients and their caregivers (Davydow *et al.*, 2009) are being increasingly recognised in the ICU setting. Current literature describes the use of non-pharmacological interventions such as hydration, music therapy and cognitive stimulation to assist in delirium prevention. However, the majority of the literature is in non-ICU patients. It is reasonable to assume that patients in the ICU are at an inherently higher risk of delirium due to their exposure to risk factors such as mechanical ventilation. There is currently a relative void of evidence for what non-pharmacological interventions are the most impactful in this population (Rivosecchi *et al.*, 2016). Additionally, if frailty increases delirium risk, this might also be included in procedures for obtaining informed consent.

The state of nutrition may be a significant predisposing risk factor for development of delirium (Rudolph *et al.*, 2009). Conversely, the occurrence of delirium in a vulnerable older patient can stress at-risk fat and protein stores and potentiate sarcopenia. Nutritional requirements in the delirious intensive care patient care routinely addressed through tube or parenteral feeding regimes, though these regimens often fail to meet the patient's caloric needs. Delirious patients outside of the ICU setting are particularly vulnerable to underfeeding and weight loss, none more so than in the nursing home setting (Culp and Cacchione, 2008). Even though frailty is associated with a higher risk of functional decline and worsening disability after an acute illness, the mechanism through which frailty influences negative functional outcomes in delirium remains to be elucidated (Chew *et al.*, 2017).

References

Abdelhafiz AH, McNicholas E, Sinclair AJ. (2016). Hypoglycemia, frailty and dementia in older people with diabetes: reciprocal relations and clinical implications. *J Diabetes Complications*. November–December; 30(8): 1548–54. doi:10.1016/j.jdiacomp. 2016.07.027. Epub 2016 July 27.

Abdullah HR, Lien VP, Ong HK, Er PL, Hao Y, Khan SA, Liu CW. (2017). Protocol for a single-centre, randomised controlled study of a preoperative rehabilitation bundle in the frail and elderly undergoing abdominal surgery. *BMJ Open*. August 4; 7(8):e016815. doi:10.1136/bmjopen-2017-016815.

Amanzio M, Palermo S, Zucca M, Rosato R, Rubino E, Leotta D, Bartoli M, Rainero I. (2017). Neuropsychological correlates of pre-frailty in neurocognitive disorders: a possible role for metacognitive dysfunction and mood changes. *Front Med* (Lausanne). November 15; 4: 199. doi:10.3389/fmed.2017.00199. eCollection 2017.

Andrew MK, Freter SH, Rockwood K. (2005). Incomplete functional recovery after delirium in elderly people: a prospective cohort study. *BMC Geriatr*. March 17; 5: 5.

Athari F, Hillman KM, Frost SA. (2017). The concept of frailty in intensive care. *Aust Crit Care*. December 9. pii: S1036–7314(17)30162–5. doi:10.1016/j.aucc.2017.11.005. [Epub ahead of print].

Bellelli G, Moresco R, Panina-Bordignon P, Arosio B, Gelfi C, Morandi A, Cesari M. (2017). Is delirium the cognitive harbinger of frailty in older adults? A review about the existing evidence. *Front Med* (Lausanne). November 8; 4:188. doi:10.3389/fmed.2017.00188. eCollection 2017.

Boyle PA, Buchman AS, Wilson RS, Leurgans SE, Bennett DA. (2010). Physical frailty is associated with incident mild cognitive impairment in community-based older persons. *J Am Geriatr Soc*. 58: 248–55.

Braak H, Braak E. (1991). Neuropathological staging of Alzheimer-related changes. *Acta Neuropathol* (Berl.) 82: 239–59.

Braak H, Braak E. (1997). Frequency of stages of Alzheimer-related lesions in different age categories. *Neurobiol Aging*. 18: 351–7.

Buchman AS, Bennett DA. (2013). Cognitive frailty. *J Nutr Health Aging*. 17(9): 738–9.

Cano A. (2015). Cognitive frailty, a new target for healthy ageing. *Maturitas*. October; 82(2): 139–40. doi:10.1016/j.maturitas.2015.07.026. Epub 2015 August 1.

Cano C, Samper-Ternent R, Al Snih S, Markides K, Ottenbacher KJ. (2012). Frailty and cognitive impairment as predictors of mortality in older Mexican Americans. *J Nutr Health Aging*. 16: 142–7.

Chetelat G, Baron JC. (2003). Early diagnosis of Alzheimer's disease: contribution of structural neuroimaging. *NeuroImage*. 18: 525–41.

Chew J, Lim WS, Chong MS, Ding YY, Tay L. (2017). Impact of frailty and residual subsyndromal delirium on 1-year functional recovery: a prospective cohort study. *Geriatr Gerontol Int*. June 22. doi: 10.1111/ggi.13108. [Epub ahead of print].

Cooper Z, Rogers SO Jr, Ngo L, Guess J, Schmitt E, Jones RN, Ayres DK, Walston JD, Gill TM, Gleason LJ, Inouye SK, Marcantonio ER. (2016). Comparison of frailty measures as predictors of outcomes after orthopedic surgery. *J Am Geriatr Soc*. December; 64(12): 2464–71. doi:10.1111/jgs.14387. Epub 2016 November 1.

Crocco EA, Loewenstein DA. (2005). Psychiatric aspects of mild cognitive impairment. *Curr Psychiatry Rep.* 7: 32–6.

Culp KR, Cacchione PZ. (2008). Nutritional status and delirium in long-term care elderly individuals. *Appl Nurs Res.* 21: 66–74. [PubMed: 18457745].

Cunningham C, Wilcockson DC, Campion S, Lunnon K, Perry VH. (2005). Central and systemic endotoxin challenges exacerbate the local inflammatory response and increase neuronal death during chronic neurodegeneration. *J Neurosci.* 25: 9275–84.

Dartigues JF, Amieva H. (2014). Cognitive frailty: rational and definition from an (I.A.N.A./I.A.G.G.) international consensus group. *J Nutr Health Aging.* 18(1): 95.

Dasgupta M, Rolfson DB, Stolee P, Borrie MJ, Speechley M. (2009). Frailty is associated with postoperative complications in older adults with medical problems. *Archives of Gerontology and Geriatrics.* 48(1): 78–83.

Davydow DS, Gifford JM, Desai SV, Bienvenu OJ, Needham DM. (2009). Depression in general intensive care unit survivors: a systematic review. *Intensive Care Med.* 35: 796–809.

Doig GS, Simpson F, Finfer S, Delaney A, Davies AR, Mitchell I, Dobb G. (2008). Effect of evidence-based feeding guidelines on mortality of critically ill adults: a cluster randomised controlled trial. *JAMA.* 300: 2731–41.

Eamer G, Gibson JA, Gillis C, Hsu AT, Krawczyk M, MacDonald E, Whitlock R, Khadaroo RG. (2017). Surgical frailty assessment: a missed opportunity. *BMC Anesthesiol.* July 24; 17(1): 99. doi:10.1186/s12871-017-0390-7.

Eeles EM, White SV, O'Mahony SM, Bayer AJ, Hubbard RE. (2012). The impact of frailty and delirium on mortality in older inpatients. *Age Ageing.* 41(3): 412–16.

Feng L, Zin Nyunt MS, Gao Q, Feng L, Yap KB, Ng TP. (2017). Cognitive frailty and adverse health outcomes: findings from the Singapore Longitudinal Ageing Studies (SLAS). *J Am Med Dir Assoc.* March 1; 18(3): 252–8. doi:10.1016/j.jamda.2016.09.015. Epub 2016 November 9.

Fink HA, Jutkowitz E, McCarten JR, Hemmy LS, Butler M, Davila H, Ratner E, Calvert C, Barclay TR, Brasure M, Nelson VA, Kane RL. (2018). Pharmacologic interventions to prevent cognitive decline, mild cognitive impairment, and clinical Alzheimer-type dementia: a systematic review. *Ann Intern Med.* January 2; 168(1): 39–51. doi:10.7326/M17-1529. Epub 2017 December 19.

Folks DG, Freeman 3rd, AM, Sokol RS, Govier AV, Reves JG, Baker DM. (1988). Cognitive dysfunction after coronary artery bypass surgery: a case-controlled study. *Southern Medical Journal.* 81: 202–6.

Fong TG, Tulebaev SR, Inouye SK. (2009). Delirium in elderly adults: diagnosis, prevention andtment. *Nat Rev Neurol.* 5: 210–20. [PubMed: 19347026].

Ford AH. (2016). Preventing delirium in dementia: managing risk factors. *Maturitas.* October; 92: 35–40. doi:10.1016/j.maturitas.2016.07.007. Epub 2016 July 9.

Franzmeier N, Göttler J, Grimmer T, Drzezga A, Áraque-Caballero MA, Simon-Vermot L, Taylor ANW, Bürger K, Catak C, Janowitz D, Müller C, Duering M, Sorg C, Ewers M. (2017). Resting-state connectivity of the left frontal cortex to the default mode and dorsal attention network supports reserve in mild cognitive impairment. *Front Aging Neurosci.* August 7; 9: 264. doi:10.3389/fnagi.2017.00264. eCollection 2017.

Friedman J, Lussiez A, Sullivan J, Wang S, Englesbe M. (2015). Implications of sarcopenia in major surgery. *Nutr Clin Pract.* April; 30(2): 175–9. doi:10.1177/0884533615569888. Epub 2015 February 13.

Gielen S, Simm A. (2017). Frailty and cardiac rehabilitation: a long-neglected connection. *Eur J Prev Cardiol.* January 1: 2047487317707842. doi:10.1177/2047487317707842. [Epub ahead of print].

Griffiths R, Beech F, Brown A, Dhesi J, Foo I, Goodall J, Harrop-Griffiths W, Jameson J, Love N, Pappenheim K, White S. (2014). Peri-operative care of the elderly 2014. *Anaesthesia.* 69: 81–98.

Grundman M, Jack Jr., CR, Petersen RC, Kim HT, Taylor C, Datvian M *et al.*; Alzheimer's Disease Cooperative Study. (2003). Hippocampal volume is associated with memory but not nonmemory cognitive performance in patients with mild cognitive impairment. *J Mol Neurosci.* 20: 241–8.

Handoll HH, Parker PJ. (2008). Conservative versus operative treatment for hip fractures in adults. *Cochrane Database Syst Rev, Issue 3.* CD 000337. doi:10.1002/14651858. CD000337.pub2.

Harari D, Hopper A, Dhesi J, Babic-Illman G, Lockwood L, Martin F. (2007). Proactive care of older people undergoing surgery ('POPS'): designing, embedding, evaluating and funding a comprehensive geriatric assessment service for older elective surgical patients. *Age Ageing.* 36: 190–6.

Haymore JB, Patel N. (2016). Delirium in the neuro intensive care unit. *Crit Care Nurs Clin North Am.* March; 28(1): 21–35. doi:10.1016/j.cnc.2015.11.001.

Hewitt J, Moug SJ, Middleton M, Chakrabarti M, Stechman MJ, McCarthy K; Older Persons Surgical Outcomes Collaboration. (2015). Prevalence of frailty and its association with mortality in general surgery. *Am J Surg.* February; 209(2): 254–9. doi:10.1016/j. amjsurg.2014.05.022. Epub 2014 July 27.

Hii TB, Lainchbury JG, Bridgman PG. (2015). Frailty in acute cardiology: comparison of a quick clinical assessment against a validated frailty assessment tool. *Heart Lung Circ.* 24(6): 551–6. doi:10.1016/j.hlc.2014.11.024.

Inouye SK. (2006). Delirium in older persons. *N Engl J Med.* 354: 1157–65.

Inouye SK, Charpentier PA. (1996). Precipitating factors for delirium in hospitalized elderly persons: predictive model and interrelationship with baseline vulnerability. *JAMA.* 275(11): 852–7.

Inouye SK, Westendorp RG, Saczynski JS. (2014). Delirium in elderly people. *Lancet.* March 8; 383(9920): 911–22. doi:10.1016/S0140-6736(13)60688-1. Epub 2013 August 28.

Joosten E, Demuynck M, Detroyer E, Milisen K. (2014). Prevalence of frailty and its ability to predict in hospital delirium, falls, and 6-month mortality in hospitalized older patients. *BMC Geriatr.* January 6; 14: 1. doi:10.1186/1471-2318-14-1.

Kantarci K, Jack Jr., CR. (2003). Neuroimaging in Alzheimer's disease: an evidence-based review. *Neuroimaging Clin N Am.* 13: 197–209.

Kelaiditi E, Cesari M, Canevelli M, van Kan GA, Ousset PJ, Gillette-Guyonnet S, Ritz P, Duveau F, Soto ME, Provencher V, Nourhashemi F, Salvà A, Robert P, Andrieu S, Rolland Y, Touchon J, Fitten JL, Vellas B; IANA/IAGG. (2013). Cognitive frailty: rational and definition from an (IANA/IAGG) international consensus group. *J Nutr Health Aging.* September; 17(9): 726–34. doi:10.1007/s12603-013-0367-2.

Korenvain C, Famiyeh IM, Dunn I, Whitehead CR, Rochon PA, McCarthy LM. (2018). Identifying frailty in primary care: a qualitative description of family physicians' gestalt impressions of their older adult patients. *BMC Fam Pract.* May 14; 19(1): 61. doi:10.1186/ s12875-018-0743-4.

Kress JP. (2009). Clinical trials of early mobilization of critically ill patients. *Crit Care Med.* 37(10 Suppl.): S442–S447.

Laakso MP, Hallikainen M, Hanninen T, Partanen K, Soininen H. (2000). Diagnosis of Alzheimer's disease: MRI of the hippocampus vs. delayed recall. *Neuropsychologia.* 38: 579–84.

Lu J, Cao LL, Zheng CH, Li P, Xie JW, Wang JB, Lin JX, Chen QY, Lin M, Tu RH, Huang CM. (2017). The preoperative frailty versus inflammation-based prognostic score:

which is better as an objective predictor for gastric cancer patients 80 years and older? *Ann Surg Oncol.* March; 24(3): 754–62. doi:10.1245/s10434-016-5656-7. Epub 2016 November 2.

Luo XG, Ding JQ, Chen SD. (2010). Microglia in the aging brain: relevance to neurodegeneration. *Mol Neurodegener.* March 24; 5: 12. doi:10.1186/1750-1326-5-12.

MacLullich AM, Hall RJ. (2011). Who understands delirium? *Age Ageing.* 40: 412–14. [PubMed: 21636556].

Makary MA, Segev DL, Pronovost PJ, Syin D, Bandeen-Roche K, Patel P, Takenaga R, Devgan L, Holzmueller CG, Tian J, Fried LP. (2010). Frailty as a predictor of surgical outcomes in older patients. *J Am Coll Surg.* June; 210(6): 901–8. doi:10.1016/j.jamcollsurg.2010.01.028. Epub 2010 April 28.

McIsaac DI, Jen T, Mookerji N, Patel A, Lalu MM. (2017). Interventions to improve the outcomes of frail people having surgery: a systematic review. *PLoS One.* December 29; 12(12): e0190071. doi:10.1371/journal.pone.0190071. eCollection 2017.

Moller JT, Cluitmans P, Rasmussen LS, Houx P, Rasmussen H, Canet J, Rabbitt P, Jolles J, Larsen K, Hanning CD, Langeron O, Johnson T, Lauven PM, Kristensen PA, Biedler A, van Beem H, Fraidakis O, Silverstein JH, Beneken JE, Gravenstein JS. (1998). Long-term postoperative cognitive dysfunction in the elderly ISPOCD1 study. ISPOCD investigators. International Study of Post-Operative Cognitive Dysfunction. *Lancet.* 351: 857–61.

Montero-Odasso MM, Barnes B, Speechley M, Muir Hunter SW, Doherty TJ, Duque G, Gopaul K, Sposato LA, Casas-Herrero A, Borrie MJ, Camicioli R, Wells JL. (2016). Disentangling cognitive-frailty: results from the Gait and Brain Study. *Gerontol A Biol Sci Med Sci.* November; 71(11): 1476–82. Epub 2016 March 16.

Morris JC, Storandt M, Miller JP, McKeel DW, Price JL, Rubin EH et al. (2001). Mild cognitive impairment represents early-stage Alzheimer's disease. *Arch. Neurol.* 58: 397–405.

Moug SJ, Stechman M, McCarthy K, Pearce L, Myint PK, Hewitt J; Older Persons Surgical Outcomes Collaboration. (2016). Frailty and cognitive impairment: unique challenges in the older emergency surgical patient. *Ann R Coll Surg Engl.* March; 98(3): 165–9. doi:10.1308/rcsann.2016.0087.

Oakland K, Nadler R, Cresswell L, Jackson D, Coughlin PA. (2016). Systematic review and meta-analysis of the association between frailty and outcome in surgical patients. *Ann R Coll Surg Engl.* February; 98(2): 80–5. doi:10.1308/rcsann.2016.0048. Epub 2016 January 7.

Panza F, D'Introno A, Colacicco AM, Capurso C, Parigi AD, Capurso SA, Caselli RJ, Pilotto A, Scafato E, Capurso A, Solfrizzi V. (2006). Cognitive frailty: predemedia syndrome and vascular risk factors. *Neurobiol Aging.* July; 27(7): 933–40. Epub 2005 July 14.

Partridge JS, Harari D, Dhesi JK. (2012). Frailty in the older surgical patient: a review. *Age Ageing.* March; 41(2): 142–7. doi:10.1093/ageing/afr182.

Pendlebury ST, Lovett NG, Smith SC, Wharton R, Rothwell PM. (2017). Delirium risk stratification in consecutive unselected admissions to acute medicine: validation of a susceptibility score based on factors identified externally in pooled data for use at entry to the acute care pathway. *Age Ageing.* March 1; 46(2): 226–31. doi:10.1093/ageing/afw198.

Pennanen C, Kivipelto M, Tuomainen S, Hartikainen P, Hanninen T, Laakso MP et al. (2004). Hippocampus and entorhinal cortex in mild cognitive impairment and early AD. *Neurobiol Aging.* 25: 303–10.

Petersen RC, Doody R, Kurz A, Mohs RC, Morris JC. (2001). Current concepts in mild cognitive impairment. *Arch Neurol.* 58: 1985–92.

Petersen RC, Smith GE, Waring SC, Ivnik RJ, Tangalos EG. (1999). Mild cognitive impairment: clinical characterization and outcome. *Arch Neurol.* 56: 303–8.

Pilotto A, Rengo F, Marchionni N, Sancarlo D, Fontana A, Panza F, Ferrucci L; FIRI-SIGG Study Group. (2012). Comparing the prognostic accuracy for all-cause mortality of frailty instruments: a multicentre 1-year follow-up in hospitalized older patients. *PloS One.* 7(1): e29090. doi:10.1371/journal.pone.0029090. Epub 2012 January 11.

Psutka SP, Carrasco A, Schmit GD, Moynagh MR, Boorjian SA, Frank I, Stewart SB, Thapa P, Tarrell RF, Cheville JC, Tollefson MK. (2014). Sarcopenia in patients with bladder cancer undergoing radical cystectomy: impact on cancer-specific and all-cause mortality. *Cancer.* 120(18): 2910–18. doi:10.1002/cncr.28798.

Quinlan N, Marcantonio ER, Inouye SK, Gill TM, Kamholz B, Rudolph JL. (2011). Vulnerability: the crossroads of frailty and delirium. *J Am Geriatr Soc.* November; 59(Suppl. 2): S262–8. doi:10.1111/j.1532-5415.2011.03674.x.

Revenig LM, Canter DJ, Taylor MD, Tai C, Sweeney JF, Sarmiento JM *et al.* (2013). Too frail for surgery? Initial results of a large multidisciplinary prospective study examining preoperative variables predictive of poor surgical outcomes. *Journal of the American College of Surgeons.* 217(4): 665–70.e1.

Richardson SJ, Davis DHJ, Stephan B, Robinson L, Brayne C, Barnes L, Parker S, Allan LM. (2017). Protocol for the Delirium and Cognitive Impact in Dementia (DECIDE) study: a nested prospective longitudinal cohort study. *BMC Geriatr.* April 28; 17(1): 98. doi:10.1186/s12877-017-0479-3.

Rivosecchi RM, Kane-Gill SL, Svec S, Campbell S, Smithburger PL. (2016). The implementation of a nonpharmacologic protocol to prevent intensive care delirium. *J Crit Care.* February; 31(1): 206–11. doi:10.1016/j.jcrc.2015.09.031. Epub 2015 October 17.

Robinson TN, Eiseman B, Wallace JI, Church SD, McFann KK, Pfister SM, Sharp TJ, Moss M. (2009). Redefining geriatric preoperative assessment using frailty, disability and co-morbidity. *Ann Surg.* September; 250(3): 449–55. doi:10.1097/SLA.0b013e3181b45598.

Robinson TN, Wu DS, Stiegmann GV, Moss M. (2011). Frailty predicts increased hospital and six-month healthcare cost following colorectal surgery in older adults. *Am J Surg.* 2020(5): 511–14.

Rosczyk HA, Sparkman NL, Johnson RW. (2008). Neuroinflammation and cognitive function in aged mice following minor surgery. *Experimental Gerontology.* 43: 840–6.

Rudolph JL, Jones RN, Levkoff SE, Rockett C, Inouye SK, Sellke FW *et al.* (2009). Derivation and validation of a preoperative prediction rule for delirium after cardiac surgery. *Circulation.* 119: 229–36. [PubMed: 19118253].

Saczynski JS, Marcantonio ER, Quach L, Fong TG, Gross A, Inouye SK, Jones RN. (2012). Cognitive trajectories after postoperative delirium. *N Engl J Med.* 367: 30–9.

Salisbury LG, Merriweather JL, Walsh TS. (2010). The development and feasibility of a ward-based physiotherapy and nutritional rehabilitation package for people experiencing critical illness. *Clin Rehabil.* 24: 489–500.

Satz P. (1993). Brain reserve capacity on symptom onset after brain injury: a formulation and review of evidence for threshold theory. *Neuropsychology.* 7: 273–95.

Schweickert WD, Pohlman MC, Pohlman AS, Nigos C, Pawlik AJ, Esbrook CL *et al.* (2009). Early physical and occupational therapy in mechanically ventilated, critically ill patients: a randomised controlled trial. *Lancet.* 373(9678): 1874–82.

Shaw PJ, Bates D, Cartlidge NE, French JM, Heaviside D, Julian DG, Shaw DA. (1987). Long-term intellectual dysfunction following coronary artery bypass graft surgery: a six month follow-up study. *Q J Med.* March; 62(239): 259–68.

Shimada H, Makizako H, Lee S, Doi T, Lee S, Tsutsumimoto K, Harada K, Hotta R, Bae S, Nakakubo S, Harada K, Suzuki T. (2016). Impact of cognitive frailty on daily activities in older persons. *J Nutr Health Aging*. 20(7): 729–35. doi:10.1007/s12603-016-0685-2.

Siddiqi N, Harrison JK, Clegg A, Teale EA, Young J, Taylor J, Simpkins SA. (2016). Interventions for preventing delirium in hospitalised non-ICU patients. *Cochrane Database Syst Rev*. March 11; 3: CD005563. doi:10.1002/14651858.CD005563.pub3.

Sperling RA, Aisen PS, Beckett LA, Bennett D, Craft S, Fagan A *et al*. (2011). Toward defining the preclinical stages of Alzheimer's disease: recommendations from the National Institute on Aging-Alzheimer's Association workgroups on diagnostic guidelines for Alzheimer's disease. *Alzheimers Dement*. 7: 280–92.

Stern, Y. (2002). What is cognitive reserve? Theory and research application of the reserve concept. *J Int Neuropsychol Soc*. 8(3): 448–60.

Stevens JA. (2005). Falls among older adults: risk factors and prevention strategies. *J Safety Res*. 36(4): 409–11.

Stoicea N, Baddigam R, Wajahn J, Sipes AC, Arias-Morales CE, Gastaldo N, Bergese SD. (2016). The gap between clinical research and standard of care: a review of frailty assessment scales in perioperative surgical settings. *Front Public Health*. July 21; 4: 150. doi:10.3389/fpubh.2016.00150. eCollection 2016.

Streit WJ. (2006). Microglial senescence: does the brain's immune system have an expiration date? *Trends Neurosci*. 29: 506–10.

Teale EA, Young JR. (2015). Multicomponent delirium prevention interventions: not as effective as NICE suggest? *Age and Ageing*. 44(6): 915–17.

Terry RD. (2000). Cell death or synaptic loss in Alzheimer's disease. *J Neuropathol Exp Neurol*. 59: 1118–19.

Torrance AD, Powell SL, Griffiths EA. (2015). Emergency surgery in the elderly: challenges and solutions. *Open Access Emerg Med*. September 8; 7: 55–68. doi:10.2147/OAEM.S68324. eCollection 2015.

Velanovich V, Antoine H, Swartz A, Peters D, Rubinfeld I. (2013). Accumulating deficits model of frailty and postoperative mortality and morbidity: its application to a national database. *Journal of Surgical Research*. 183: 104–10.

Verloo H, Goulet C, Morin D, von Gunten A. (2016). Association between frailty and delirium in older adult patients discharged from hospital. *Clin Interv Aging*. 11: 55–63.

Watt J, Tricco AC, Talbot-Hamon C, Pham B, Rios P, Grudniewicz A, Wong C, Sinclair D, Straus SE. (2018). Identifying older adults at risk of harm following elective surgery: a systematic review and meta-analysis. *BMC Med*. January 12; 16(1): 2. doi:10.1186/s12916-017-0986-2.

Wolf H, Hensel A, Kruggel F, Riedel-Heller SG, Arendt T, Wahlund LO *et al*. (2004). Structural correlates of mild cognitive impairment. *Neurobiol Aging*. 25: 913–24.

5

SARCOPENIA AND FRAILTY

Aim

Sarcopenia is of special interest as it describes a specific condition where translationary research might produce benefits and outcomes for clinical patients. It is also a case where elucidating with precision the factors which make sarcopenia better or worse, through assets or deficits, will be of great help for the future.

Introduction

Sarcopenia is now firmly on the agenda for research on ageing, and now, arguably, needs to be recognised in routine clinical practice (Sayer, 2014). Sarcopenia appears to be significantly associated with higher risk of mortality among sub-groups of older patients with limited mobility and impaired functional status, independently of age and other clinical variables (Pourhassan *et al.*, 2018).

The gap between the demand of effective intervention strategies and the availability of medical pathways specifically dedicated to older adults can result in inappropriate use of resources and escalating healthcare expenditures (Marzetti *et al.*, 2016). Skeletal muscle has a number of critical functions. It is the largest reserve of protein in the body, and during periods of stress, under-nutrition or starvation, it provides a continuous supply of amino acids to maintain protein synthetic rate in other vital tissues. Skeletal muscle is the primary site of glucose disposal, and diminished muscle mass may play a role in impaired glucose metabolism in patients with insulin resistance and type 2 diabetes (e.g. DeFronzo and Tripathy, 2009).

More than 600 skeletal muscles of the human body constitute 45–55 per cent of the total body mass, being muscular mass, mostly located in the lower limbs, and change significantly in size and function with ageing. These changes may lead to decreased physical performance, decline of strength, mobility impairment, falls and disability (Frontera *et al.*, 2005). Distinctions among senescence, ageing and disease blur for the late-life chronic diseases and conditions because, in addition to disease processes, many chronic degenerative diseases are phenotypic manifestations of senescing DNA, organelles, cells and organs (Crews, 2007). Although the prolongation of life remains an important public health goal, the preservation of adequate levels of function and independence into late life is a fundamental requisite for assuring sustainability of social and healthcare systems (Landi *et al.*, 2017). Today sarcopenia is increasingly being recognised as the biological substrate underlying the development of physical frailty, and a key mechanism leading to the negative outcomes of frailty such as mobility disability and physical dependency (Del Signore and Roubenoff, 2017).

Skeletal muscle protein turnover is a complex regulated process.

Prevalence

Prevalence estimates for sarcopenia vary widely in different clinical settings, reflecting divergence in the approaches used for definition. Thus, rates of between 1 and 29 per cent have been reported in community-dwelling populations and of 14–33 per cent in residents requiring long-term care (Cruz-Jentoft *et al.*, 2014). On average, it is estimated that 5–13 per cent of elderly people aged 60–70 years are affected by sarcopenia. The numbers increase to 11–50 per cent for those aged 80 or above.

History

'Sarcopenia' (from the Greek *sarx*, 'flesh', and *penia*, 'loss') identifies the age-associated loss of muscle mass and function. The term was formally coined nearly 30 years ago by Rosenberg (1989), who remarked that 'No single feature of age-related decline (is) more striking than the decline in lean body mass (which) affects ambulation, mobility, energy intake, overall nutrient intake and status, independence, and breathing.' While sarcopenia is a highly prevalent condition with enormous personal and societal costs, a unique operational definition has not yet been achieved. As a consequence, no definite treatment guidelines are presently available (Reginster *et al.*, 2016).

Definition and identification of sarcopenia

Sarcopenia is defined as the combination of wasting muscle mass and decreased physical performance that occurs as people age (Fielding *et al.*, 2011; Cruz-Jentoft *et al.*, 2010).

Arguably, there is no guidance to help clinicians identify older adults with clinically meaningful low muscle mass or weakness. Low lean muscle mass (LLM), assessed using intelligent dual energy X-ray absorptiometry, is a component of the frailty syndrome but not universally present. Indeed, LLM and frailty are associated and partly overlapped; future research including longitudinal studies should perhaps look at combining LLM and frailty measures in preventing disability (Fougère *et al.*, 2018).

Furthermore, development of novel sarcopenia therapies is compromised not only due to the difficulty in identifying participants for clinical trials, but also because there are no validated, clinically appropriate endpoints for assessment of treatment efficacy (McLean and Kiel, 2015).

Despite promising advances in evaluating muscle mass and strength, the multiple mechanisms at the basis of sarcopenia have not yet been fully characterised; nevertheless, a series of biomarkers may be found in both tissue and blood samples (Kalinkovich and Livshits, 2015). The lack of a univocal operational definition of sarcopenia represents a major limitation in the field. It is now widely acknowledged that sarcopenia encompasses both quantitative (i.e. mass) and qualitative (i.e. strength and/or function) declines of skeletal muscle (Calvani *et al.*, 2015). Yet, depending on the tools used for the assessment of muscle mass and function and the reference values considered, the resulting phenotypes are only partly overlapping (Scott *et al.*, 2014).

A wide range of techniques can be used to assess muscle mass. Cost, availability and ease of use can determine whether the techniques are better suited to clinical practice or are more useful for research. No one technique subserves all requirements, but dual energy X-ray absorptiometry could be considered as a reference standard (but not a gold standard) for measuring LLM based on feasibility, accuracy, safety and low cost (Buckinx *et al.*, 2018).

Sarcopenia is essentially present when there is a less-than-expected muscle mass in an individual of a specified age, gender and race (Baumgartner and Waters, 2006). Baumgartner was the first to provide a working definition for sarcopenia. He used an 'index of relative muscle mass', which was defined as appendicular skeletal muscle mass, measured by dual-energy X-ray absorptiometry (DEXA), divided by the square of stature. Sarcopenia was diagnosed if an individual's muscle mass lay more than two standard deviations below the mean muscle mass of normal, healthy young men and women younger than age 30 (Baumgartner *et al.*, 1998). The widespread use of magnetic resonance imaging and computed tomography scan for the non-invasive assessment of muscle mass is limited in primary care settings by difficulties in access, costs, the lack of portable equipment and the requirement of highly specialised personnel (Beaudart *et al.*, 2016).

The **Foundation for the National Institutes of Health (FNIH) Sarcopenia Project** provides a further step toward a consensus definition of sarcopenia among older people by including data from nine studies of community-dwelling older individuals to determine a recommended set of clinically relevant criteria incorporating a large, diverse and well-characterised set of populations (Studenski *et al.*, 2014). Recommendations for further analyses by the FNIH consortium are to evaluate their cut-off points in additional studies to determine whether they identify groups of older adults who are likely to benefit from interventions designed to maintain or improve outcomes.

The **Foundation for the Institutes of Health (FNIH) Biomarkers Consortium** have published cut-off points for grip strength and appendicular lean mass divided by body mass index (ALMBMI). To do this, they pooled data from nine U.S. and European studies of community-dwelling older people and calculated the cut-off points that best identified individuals with a gait speed of less than 0.8 m/s.

Some of the advantages and disadvantages of methods used to measure muscle mass and strength are shown in Table 5.1.

Sarcopenia and frailty are mutual risk factors, and both conditions can co-occur within a single individual. The terms 'sarcopenia' and 'frailty' are often used interchangeably in clinical practice; however, both have a different construct and require a different therapeutic approach. A diagnosis of sarcopenia remains a relatively rare case. To date, there is not a unique, well-accepted, validated and/or standardised way to identify the presence of sarcopenia in an older person. This deficiency significantly affects each operative definition and leads to different results. Sarcopenia can be quantified by indexing fat-free mass (FFM) or appendicular FFM both from DEXA by height squared, fat mass or total mass (Chumlea et al., 2011). DEXA is a well established, low-radiation technique used to assess body composition and provides reproducible estimates of appendicular skeletal lean mass (LeVine et al., 2000). But even if the diagnosis is reached, the treatment of sarcopenia remains challenging. Many different approaches have been pursued, but exercise and physical activity are important considerations for both sarcopenia prophylaxis and sarcopenia management (von Haehling et al., 2010).

A rapid screening test for sarcopenia has been developed – the '**SARC-F**'. This screen for sarcopenia has been validated in three separate populations (St. Louis African American Study, Baltimore Longitudinal Study and National Health and Nutrition Examination Survey (NHANES)), as well as in two studies in China. It appears to have equivalent predictive capacity to a number of the more complex definitions for sarcopenia (Morley, 2016). This requires the development of better screening tools to detect and assess sarcopenia in the elderly, and of robust biomarkers and new treatment options (Calvari et al., 2018). Sarcopenia is very often not noticeable in earlier phases but becomes more apparent once a critical event such as a fall has occurred or disability has set in. While it is possible to preserve skeletal muscle mass in older age, it is extremely challenging to regain substantial quantities once the loss has occurred. Therefore, a screening strategy to a larger population in the community that allows for early detection is important (Yu et al., 2016). Finally, in a recent study, Kashani and colleagues (2017) have reported a '**sarcopenia index**' (SI) [(serum creatinine value/cystatin C value) × 100] as a novel blood test to approximate muscle mass. These authors proposed that their SI is a potentially objective measure for estimating muscle mass that is non-invasive and less expensive.

Sarcopenia and frailty

Both the concepts of frailty and sarcopenia are evolving, and there is still no full consensus on where to fit each of them in usual clinical practice, or on how to use either to prevent or slow down disability.

TABLE 5.1 Advantages and disadvantages of methods that can be used to measure muscle mass and strength

Measurement methods	Advantages	Disadvantages
Muscle mass		
DXA	Three-component model combining protein and minerals into 'solids'	Unable to evaluated intramuscular fat
	Wide availability; high precision; low radiation; regional and whole-body measurements of the three components	Modest cost, size (weight and height) limitations. Cannot specifically discern skeletal muscle mass and quality as can CT and MRI
Anthropometry	Simple to measure	Lacks precision and prone to overestimation
	Non-invasive and inexpensive	Inter-observer variation may occur
	Applicable in large surveys	Training required
Bio-electrical impedance	Easy to use in both research and clinical settings	Lack of standardised methodology
	Variable instrument cost, safe, potentially portable, useful for long-term monitoring and longitudinal studies	Measurements sensitive to subject conditions such as hydration and recent activity
		Instrument predictions may be population-specific
Imaging		
MRI and CT	More sensitive to small changes than DXA	Subject size limitations
	High resolution	
Muscle strength		
Isometric/isokinetic	Recognised gold standard for measuring muscle strength	Cost and availability of equipment
Grip strength	Simple to measure	Variation in methodology makes comparisons between studies difficult
		Use of standard Jamar dynamometer may be difficult for some patients

Source: adapted from Heymsfield *et al.*, 2015, p. 357, Table 1; and Shaw *et al.*, 2017, p. 233, Table 2.

Note

Methods that are commonly used in research and clinical settings are shown in italics.

One model of frailty starts with sarcopenia and reduced expenditure of energy; this leads to weight loss, weakness, exhaustion and low levels of physical ability, i.e. frailty (Crews, 2007). Frailty, sarcopenia and immunosenescence are commonly described in older adults but are not unique to ageing. There is evidence that all three conditions are reversible and all three appear to share common inflammatory drivers. It is unclear whether frailty, sarcopenia and immunesenescence are separate entities that co-occur due to coincidental or potentially confounding factors, or whether they are more intimately linked by the same underlying cellular mechanisms (Wilson *et al.*, 2017). In light of the growing body of data implicating senescent cells in age-related disease and frailty, a number of strategies are being considered to mitigate these deleterious effects. First, the cell stresses and signaling pathways that lead to senescence-associated growth arrest could be targeted by therapeutic interventions (LeBrasseur *et al.*, 2015).

Sarcopenia may lead to frailty, but not all patients with sarcopenia are frail – it is estimated that sarcopenia is about twice as common as frailty (Von Haehling *et al.*, 2010). Frailty is associated with a 'pro-inflammatory state', which has been characterised by elevated levels of systemic inflammatory biomarkers, but has not been related to the number of co-existing chronic diseases associated with inflammation (Chang *et al.*, 2012). Sarcopenia can be categorised as 'primary' (age-related) or 'secondary' (disease-related) sarcopenia. Disease-related sarcopenia is associated with advanced organ failure and chronic inflammatory diseases, such as chronic heart failure and chronic kidney disease secondary to cardiovascular diseases (Cruz-Jentoft *et al.*, 2010). For example, particularly in patients with CHF, sarcopenia is a major factor of reduced quality of life, as well as in the progression to frailty and cardiac cachexia (Springer *et al.*, 2017). Therefore, more basic research, as well as clinical trials, are urgently needed.

An overview of pathways to adverse outcomes is shown in Figure 5.1.

Both frailty models have an overlap in the physical component. In this regard, muscle plays an important role.

It was once decided that 'sarcopenia with limited mobility' might be an acceptable term to define persons with a need for therapeutic interventions. This is a specific condition with clear loss of muscle mass and a clear target for intervention. As such, it differs from the more general concept of frailty. The definition is based on consensus and may change as additional data become available. 'Sarcopenia with limited mobility' is a syndrome, not a disease. It is defined as a person with muscle loss whose walking speed is equal to or less than 1 m/s or who walks less than 400 m during a 6-minute walk (Morley *et al.*, 2011). Although frailty is a more complex problem that includes physical, functional, mental and social aspects, in our view sarcopenia can be considered as being a key pathway between frailty and disability (Cruz-Jentoft and Michel, 2013).

Sarcopenia is one of the most pathophysiological characteristics of frailty. Pattison and colleagues found that in sarcopenic skeletal muscle from old rats, 7 per cent of the genes that were differentially expressed against non-sarcopenic muscle from young rats were related to stress/antioxidant responses (Pattison *et al.*, 2003).

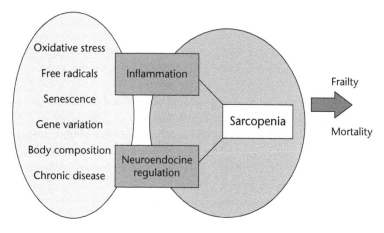

FIGURE 5.1 Possible pathway

Source: adapted from Figure 1, p. 676 of Bauer JM, Sieber CC. (2008). Sarcopenia and frailty: a clinician's controversial point of view. *Exp Gerontol.* July; 43(7): 674–8. doi:10.1016/j. exger.2008.03.007. Epub 2008 March 25.

Biomarkers of oxidative stress have also been associated with frailty in the Framingham Offspring Study, suggesting oxidative stress as the underlying mechanism contributing to frailty (Liu *et al.*, 2016). Whether targeted interventions at preventing functional decline may result in an improved pro- and anti-inflammatory balance, regardless of age of the patient, remains to be established (Van Epps *et al.*, 2016).

Introduction to risk factors for sarcopenia

Several risks factors in combination may contribute to the development of sarcopenia (Figure 5.2).

Simplifying, the risk factors for the development of sarcopenia can be grouped into different categories (Marzetti *et al.*, 2017):

A *Personal factors*. It is well established that age per se and gender impact the prevalence of sarcopenia. Furthermore, early-life events, including low birth weight, increase the risk of sarcopenia in later life, and various genetic characteristics influence muscle metabolism and turnover over the course of life.

B *Hormonal factors and inflammation*. Derangements of several hormonal pathways (e.g. testosterone, oestrogens, growth hormone, insulin-like growth factor-1) have been described with ageing and are associated with declining muscle mass. Chronic low-grade (sub-clinical) inflammation, a hallmark of the ageing process, is also involved in the pathogenesis of sarcopenia.

Mitochondrial dysfunction in myocytes is thought to be a major contributor to muscle loss with ageing. Age-related sarcopenia has also been associated with altered mitochondrial morphology, as illustrated by the appearance of enlarged and depolarised mitochondria with aberrant mitochondrial cristae formation (Navratil *et al.*, 2008).

C   *Lifestyle habits*. Lifestyle choices, including decreases in food intake and particularly protein intake, sedentary behaviour or reduced physical activity over the life course, alcohol abuse and tobacco use, have all been associated with a high risk of sarcopenia. Furthermore, protracted bed rest and immobility cause weight loss and are responsible for dramatic muscle loss in older adults.

D   *Chronic health conditions*. Many long-lasting health conditions (including cognitive impairment or dementia, mood disturbances, diabetes and end-stage organ diseases) are associated with sarcopenia. There has been discussion in the literature regarding the effects of chronic diseases in accelerating sarcopenia progression, with mixed opinions whether disease directly contributes to sarcopenia per se (Buford *et al.*, 2010; Dardevet *et al.*, 2012).

It has been demonstrated that '**inflamm–ageing**' is considered as a significant contributor to age-related muscle wasting process (Toth *et al.*, 2006; Visser *et al.*, 2002) (see Chapter 1). Inflamm–ageing supports the development and progression of age-related diseases with an inflammatory basis, such as osteoporosis, neurodegeneration, atherosclerosis, insulin resistance and sarcopenia (Shaw *et al.*, 2010). Age-associated changes to the immune system (both immunesenescence, the

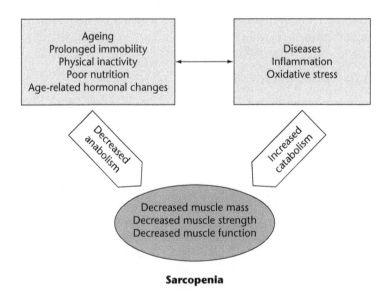

Sarcopenia

FIGURE 5.2   Major risk factors for sarcopenia

Source: redrawn from Figure 1, p. 12 of Marzetti E, Calvani R, Tosato M, Cesari M, Di Bari M, Cherubini A, Collamati A, D'Angelo E, Pahor M, Bernabei R, Landi F; SPRINTT Consortium. (2017). Sarcopenia: an overview. *Aging Clin Exp Res*. February; 29(1): 11–17. doi:10.1007/s40520-016-0704-5. Epub 2017 February 2.

decline in immune function with ageing, and inflamm-ageing, a state of chronic inflammation) have been suggested as contributors to sarcopenia and frailty, but a direct causative role remains to be established. Frailty, sarcopenia and immunesenescence are commonly described in older adults but are not unique to ageing (Wilson et al., 2017). The mechanism by which increased lymphocyte counts are positively correlated with better muscular strength and higher physical activity in older women is likely to be complex; however, increased lymphocyte counts have been positively associated with physical exercise in young people (Nielsen, 2003; Pedersen and Toft, 2000).

Pathophysiology of sarcopenia

Studies looking at the histological changes in muscle fibres reveal that sarcopenia predominantly effects the type II (fast-twitch) muscle fibres, whereas type I (slow-twitch) fibres are much less affected. The size of type II fibres can be reduced by up to 50 per cent in sarcopenia. However, such reductions are only moderate when compared with overall reductions in muscle mass (Dhillon and Hasni, 2017). Treatment of sarcopenia may be focused on maintaining or increasing muscle mass and strength by combining exercise and adequate protein intake, whereas frailty may require a focus on the underlying diverse pathophysiology of the different domains. Furthermore, prevalence rates of sarcopenia and frailty are highly dependent on the used definition (Reijnierse et al., 2016). Mechanisms involved in sarcopenia are actively being investigated and include intrinsic as well as extrinsic factors, such as deficient satellite cell recruitment, contraction-induced injury, loss of neuronal innervation, endocrine changes and an increase in oxidative stress (Dupont-Versteegden, 2005). Markers of oxidative damage have been examined in tissues of many species and it is apparent that all tissues, including skeletal muscle, of old organisms contain greater oxidative damage to lipids, DNA and proteins in comparison with those found in younger organisms (e.g. Vasilaki et al., 2006).

The pathophysiology of sarcopenia is complex and at present there is no concept that integrates all the potential causal factors in one model (Bauer et al., 2008). The molecular events that occur in muscle during sarcopenia are not well understood. Because muscle mass is determined by the net relationship between protein synthesis and breakdown, sarcopenia must be due to a relative decrease in protein synthesis, a relative increase in protein degradation or a combination of both (Kimball et al., 2004). With respect to apoptosis, skeletal muscle is a unique tissue, because muscle cells, or myofibres, are one of three cell types, along with osteoclasts and cytotrophoblasts, that are multinucleated. This aspect of skeletal muscle has led to the concept of the 'myonuclear domain', which is defined as the theoretical amount of cytoplasm supported by a single muscle fibre nucleus, or myonucleus (protein/DNA) (Cheek, 1985). Features of sarcopenia include: decreased muscle mass and cross-sectional area; infiltration of muscle by fat and connective tissue; decrease of type II fibre size and number, but also of type I fibres; accumulation of internal nuclei, ring fibres and ragged fibres; disarrangement of myofilaments and Z-lines;

proliferation of the sarcoplasmic reticulum and t-tubular system; accumulation of lipofuscin and nemaline rod structures; and decreased number of motor units (Kamel, 2003).

Various mechanisms have been put forth to explain the change in total muscle mass observed including: (1) a lack of regular physical activity ('*use it or lose it*'); (2) a change in protein metabolism (a deficit between protein synthesis versus degradation); (3) alterations in the endocrine milieu (decrease in growth hormone and testosterone and an increase in cortisol and cytokines); (4) a loss of neuromuscular function (denervation versus re-innervation); (5) altered gene expression; and (6) apoptosis. Other factors may also contribute in part to sarcopenia (Marcell, 2003). Altered neuromuscular communication during ageing is receiving increasing attention as a potential cause of sarcopenia (Pannérec *et al.*, 2016). Defects in the neuromuscular system have been demonstrated during ageing in both rodents and humans.

The 'Sarcopenia and Physical fRailty IN older people: multicomponenT Treatment strategies' project

The '**Sarcopenia and Physical fRailty IN older people: multicomponenT Treatment strategies**' (SPRINTT) project has been designed to produce significant advancements in the management of older persons with physical frailty and sarcopenia (PF&S) by promoting a consensus among academia, regulators, industry and patients' representatives over: (1) a clear operationalisation of frailty; (2) the identification of a precise target population with unmet medical needs; (3) the evaluation and validation of a new methodology for implementing in Europe preventive and therapeutic strategies among frail elders at risk of disability; (4) the definition of an experimental setting serving as template for regulatory purposes and pharmaceutical investigations; and (5) the identification of biomarkers and health technology solutions to be implemented in clinical practice (Bernabei *et al.*, 2017).

The '**PF&S condition**' is defined by the co-occurrence of low muscle mass (according to the cut-off points recommended by the Foundation for the National Institute of Health Sarcopenia Project (Cawthon *et al.*, 2014) and reduced physical performance, operationalised as a summary score on the Short Physical Performance Battery (Guralnik *et al.*, 1994) between 3 and 9.

Older adults with PF&S are randomised to either a multicomponent intervention (MCI), involving structured physical activity, nutritional counselling/dietary intervention, and an information and communication technology (ICT) intervention, or a Healthy Aging Lifestyle Education programme (Marzetti *et al.*, 2015). The physical activity programme has been taken and modified from the Lifestyle Interventions and Independence for Elders study (Pahor *et al.*, 2014), given its full safety profile and efficacy in preventing mobility disability in at-risk older persons. The nutritional component of the SPRINTT study has been designed to maximise the benefits of physical activity. Nutrition represents an important and potentially modifiable factor that impacts muscle health and the frailty status of older people (Calvani *et al.*, 2013; Michel *et al.*, 2015).

Inflammation and sarcopenia

Some studies reported that high IL-6 (interleukin 6) and CRP (C-reactive protein) levels are associated with increased risk of muscle mass and strength loss (e.g. Schaap *et al.*, 2006). CRP is an acute phase protein produced by the liver in response to elevations in IL-6. TNF-α, another cytokine, is produced mainly by macrophages, but also by lymphoid cells, mast cells, vascular endothelial cells, cardiac myocytes, adipocytes, fibroblasts and neuronal tissue. TNF-α contributes to the production of IL-6 through activation of several pathways (Singh and Newman, 2011). Moreover, some studies proved that high levels of TNF-α can increase muscle catabolism. In addition, it seems that pro-inflammatory cytokines may antagonise the anabolic effect of IGF-1, because of the development of growth hormone (GH) resistance, which decreases both circulating and muscle IGF-1 (Frost *et al.*, 2003). Low-grade elevations in levels of circulating pro-inflammatory cytokines and their receptors, such as tumour necrosis alpha (TNF-α), interleukin (IL)-6, interleukin (IL)-1 receptor antagonist (IL-1RA), soluble TNF receptors, etc., are strong independent risk factors of morbidity and mortality in the elderly (see review in De Martinis *et al.*, 2006).

The low-grade inflammation characterising the ageing process notably concurs at the pathophysiological mechanisms underlying sarcopenia. In addition, pro-inflammatory cytokines (through a variety of mechanisms, such as platelet activation and endothelial activation) may play a major role in the risk of cardiovascular events. Dysregulation of the inflammatory pathway may also affect the central nervous system and be involved in the pathophysiological mechanisms of neurodegenerative disorders (e.g. Alzheimer disease) (Michaud *et al.*, 2013). The conventional diagnostic criteria of sarcopenia include loss of skeletal muscle mass, as assessed by the '**SMI**' (skeletal muscle index), together with either weakened muscle strength, assessed by handgrip strength, or low physical performance, assessed by gait speed. Although SMI is the most important component in the diagnosis of sarcopenia, it is difficult for general physicians to measure SMI routinely because the measurement requires either bioelectrical impedance assay or dual-energy X-ray absorptiometry (Harada *et al.*, 2017).

The relation between inflammation, muscle strength and muscle mass seems to have an explanation based on the effect of inflammation on the homeostatic balance at the muscle level between protein synthesis and catabolism (Puthucheary *et al.*, 2013). Histological studies have shown that high values of serum CRP (C-reactive protein) seem to be related to reduced protein synthesis and increased protein catabolism (Zoico *et al.*, 2013). Studies have reported that inflammation can impair insulin action, modify hormone secretion and hormone receptor transduction, impair endothelial function and energy regulation and contribute to microvascular changes in the vascular system (Ahmed and Haboubi, 2010), which may contribute to muscle weakness, lack of endurance, ineffective cell metabolism and energy production, as well as impaired central nervous system control of motor movements. Results from Fragala and colleagues (2015) indicate that older women with clinically meaningful muscle weakness increased grip strength and SPPB, regardless of the presence of low lean mass, following treatment with interventions for frailty. Thus, results suggest that muscle weakness, as defined by the Foundation for the National Institutes of Health Sarcopenia Project, is a *treatable* symptom.

Bone health and sarcopenia

I first introduced the wider significance of bone health in Chapter 3. Sarcopenia results from a disproportionate decrease in synthesis and/or increase in breakdown of skeletal muscle protein (Fielding *et al.*, 2011). The genesis of both sarcopenia and osteoporosis is multifactorial. Interestingly, several factors that play a role in the origin of osteoporosis are thought to contribute to causing sarcopenia. Di Monaco and colleagues (2011) have shown a high prevalence of sarcopenia and its significant association with osteoporosis in a large sample of hip-fracture women. Data supports a research approach on preventive and treatment strategies for osteoporosis and sarcopenia targeting both bone and muscle tissue.

Nutritional interventions have also been considered but the evidence is less consistent. In particular for all the considered nutritional interventions, e.g. protein, vitamin D and antioxidant supplementation, there is a disparity between observational and experimental evidence. For example, nutritional intake declines during older age and reductions in protein intake may reduce muscle protein synthesis, both through reduced substrate availability and reduced anabolic stimulation (leucine, an amino acid, stimulates muscle protein synthesis) (Drummond and Rasmussen, 2008). In support of this hypothesis, observational evidence from longitudinal cohort studies has shown that those with the lowest protein intake have the highest rates of muscle mass decline (Houston *et al.*, 2008). However, protein supplementation studies have failed to consistently demonstrate benefit (Milne *et al.*, 2009) although investigation of the role of protein supplementation as part of a multifactorial intervention is ongoing (Romera *et al.*, 2014). Additionally, although vitamin D receptors are found on skeletal muscle cells and myopathy is a feature of vitamin D deficient diseases, low serum vitamin D is not always associated with low physical function (Annweiler *et al.*, 2009; Bolland *et al.*, 2010; Ceglia *et al.*, 2011; Bischoff-Ferrari *et al.*, 2004) in observational studies; and supplementation studies also show mixed results (Stockton *et al.*, 2011, Bischoff-Ferrari *et al.*, 2009).

Recently there has been increased evidence that osteoporosis and risk of fracture can be identified in many persons without direct measurement of bone mineral density by using the questions used in the Fracture Risk Assessment Tool (Leslie *et al.*, 2012). It has been suggested that it should be easier to identify sarcopenia using simple questions than it is to identify persons with osteoporosis. One measure has been proposed to identify sarcopenia by a set of questions, the SARC-F (Malmstrom and Morley, 2013). The association among physical inactivity, insufficient intake of energy and protein and poor muscle health in older adults suggests that physical exercise and targeted nutritional supplementation may offer substantial therapeutic gain against sarcopenia and its negative correlates (Martone *et al.*, 2017).

The environment and sarcopenia

Environmental risk factors for all three components of sarcopenia include sedentary lifestyles, adiposity and multimorbidity. The role of cigarette smoking and alcohol consumption are much less apparent than have been observed in studies of osteoporosis or cardiovascular disease (Shaw *et al.*, 2017). Nutrition has been identified as having an important influence on the development of sarcopenia; in particular, protein intake has the potential to slow the loss of muscle mass, but does not appear to be as influential as in maintaining muscle strength or physical function.

Physical activity, in particular resistance training, when performed at higher intensities, appears beneficial for muscle strength and functioning. Trials combining protein supplementation and physical activity show promising results in reducing the decline in muscle strength and function with advancing age. Progressive resistance training, performed 2–3 times per week by older people, has been shown to improve gait speed, timed get-up-and-go climbing stairs and overall muscle strength (Liu and Latham, 2009). To date, the most evidence has accrued to support exercise interventions for both frailty and sarcopenia. In particular, interventions that are delivered at least three times per week, include resistance exercise training and become progressively more challenging may be effective. One strategy is exercise training that can attenuate the process of muscle wasting by exerting anti-inflammatory and anti-oxidative effects (Bowen *et al.*, 2015). For example, progressive resistance exercise training has been shown to improve physical performance in many studies of older adults (Liu and Latham, 2009), and also to reduce the common clinical manifestations of frailty and sarcopenia, e.g. falls (Gillespie *et al.*, 2009).

The influence of **exercise** on aspects of human immune function has been examined in the short-term, such as in the minutes and hours after a single bout of exercise, after long-term exercise training interventions (e.g. months or occasionally years of regular structured exercise) or with cross-sectional and sometimes longitudinal studies (Turner, 2016). Generally acute and chronic exercise is thought to be beneficial for immune function, however a 'U-' or 'J-shaped' relationship with infection risk, that is inversely proportional to immune competence, has been proposed (Gleeson and Walsh 2012). Exercise has considerable effects on the expression of surface markers of immune cells. An acute bout of exercise induces the mobilisation of memory, naïve and senescent T-lymphocytes into the peripheral blood compartment and promotes lymphocyte apoptosis. Long-term exercise has a tendency to promote natural killer cell activity and T-lymphocytes expressing CD28 (Cao Dinh *et al.*, 2017). Recent evidence has documented a role for melatonin in reducing inflammation in muscle cells, acting specifically against these cytokines in rats and also in humans. The anti-inflammatory actions of melatonin are well-documented in numerous organs (Coto-Montes *et al.*, 2016).

Not only the lack of certain nutrients can be responsible for the onset of sarcopenia and frailty; the energy of the consumed food should also be considered. Eaten food is metabolised to provide energy for organ function and muscle activity. If intake is not sufficient to meet needs, body fat and muscle are catabolised to provide energy (Newman *et al.*, 2005). Malnutrition is one of the key pathophysiological causes of sarcopenia and it may be amenable to intervention. The prevalence of malnutrition also depends on multiple factors, including the definition used. Vanderwoude and colleagues (2012) proposed the term 'malnutrition-sarcopenia syndrome', which embodies the inherent association of both entities, highlighting their combined impact on clinical outcomes, with the aim of identifying patients and providing appropriately targeted interventions (Lardiés-Sánchez *et al.*, 2017). The intensity, duration and mode of the activity performed, as well as the nutritional status and diet (in particular daily protein intake), markedly influence skeletal muscle mass, strength and metabolism (Cartee *et al.*, 2016; Egan and Zierath, 2013). Despite the encouraging findings obtained by observational studies and small clinical trials, the effectiveness of combining physical exercise and dietary protein intervention at preventing adverse health outcomes in older adults has not yet been conclusively established.

Diabetes and sarcopenia

Diabetes is associated with an accelerated ageing process that promotes frailty. This is likely due to increased risk of sarcopenia which is linked to frailty. Other factors leading to frailty are associated diabetes complications, particularly renal impairment and dementia (Sinclair *et al.*, 2017). Among clinic patients with diabetes mellitus aged 50–90 years old, frailty and sarcopenia prevalence is high, and both syndromes are predictors of being hospitalised overnight and new ADL disability after six months (Liccini and Malmstrom, 2016). Studies of sarcopenia in older adults with diabetes are few. The Health, Aging, and Body Composition (Health ABC) Study showed that older adults with type 2 diabetes lost their knee extensor strength more rapidly than non-diabetic subjects did (Park *et al.*, 2007). In that study, diabetic patients had greater declines in muscle mass and leg muscle strength, and muscle quality was poorer in diabetic patients over three years. In addition, thigh muscle cross-sectional area also declined twice as fast in older women with diabetes than in non-diabetic subjects over six years (Park *et al.*, 2009).

Diabetes increases risk of frailty as persistent hyperglycaemia is associated with increased oxidative stress, inflammation and insulin resistance which have deleterious effects on skeletal muscle leading to sarcopenia (see Figure 5.3).

Treatment of sarcopenia

The recognition of sarcopenia and frailty as important medical syndromes has fuelled interest in the development of effective interventions and it is likely that this will be an area of change over the coming few years (Keevil and Romero-Ortuno, 2015). In particular, sarcopenia research is stimulating new drug discovery and several novel pharmaceutical interventions are being explored. These both consider new roles for existing drugs, e.g. angiotensin-converting enzyme inhibitors, and

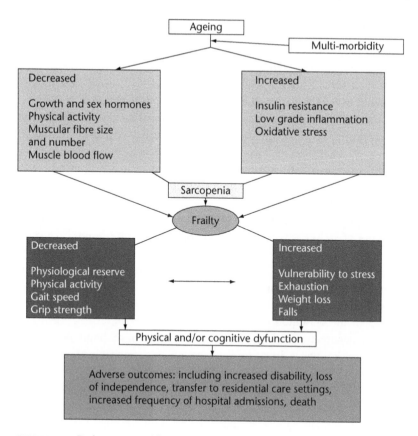

FIGURE 5.3 Pathogenesis of frailty and sarcopenia and the path to disability

Source: redrawn from Figure 1, p. 3 of Sinclair AJ, Abdelhafiz AH, Rodríguez-Mañas L. (2017). Frailty and sarcopenia: newly emerging and high impact complications of diabetes. *J Diabetes Complications*. September; 31(9): 1465–73. doi:10.1016/j.jdiacomp. 2017.05.003. Epub 2017 May 12.

the development of novel pharmaceutical agents, e.g. myostatin inhibitors (Laosa *et al.*, 2014). Selective androgen receptor molecules and ghrelin agonists are being developed to treat sarcopenia. The role of activin type IIB soluble receptors and follistatin-like 3 mimetics is less certain because of side effects (Morley and Malmstrom, 2013).

Many pharmacological agents for sarcopenia are in development. Concomitantly, in October 2016, sarcopenia received the International Classification of Diseases code M62.84, suggesting that, in the near future, family doctors and geriatricians will have the opportunity to prescribe new treatments to patients with sarcopenia. Implementation of these new drugs not only relies on evidence from research, but also the ability of the practitioner to screen and diagnose sarcopenia. Thus, assessment of sarcopenia in research but also in daily practice is becoming an important goal (Rolland *et al.*, 2017).

Sarcopenia and cachexia

Sarcopenia can be distinguished from cachexia by the more moderate degree of muscle wasting observed in the former and the absence of either associated adipose tissue wasting and/or a high inflammatory state (Morley, 2008). Ameliorating age-related skeletal muscle wasting is of high clinical importance in order to improve quality of life in the aged population, which would also reduce the socioeconomic burden of sarcopenia. Sarcopenia and cachexia represent two distinct muscle wasting diseases characterised by inflammation and oxidative stress, where specific regulating molecules associated with wasting are either activated (e.g. members of the ubiquitin proteasome system and myostatin) or repressed (e.g. insulin-like growth factor 1 and PGC-1α) (Bowen et al., 2015).

It is not always possible to distinguish cachexia from sarcopenia. Loss of muscle mass is a feature of cachexia, whereas most sarcopenic subjects are not cachectic. Persons with no weight loss, no anorexia, no measurable systemic inflammatory response may well be sarcopenic. Sarcopenia may be accelerated after an acute inflammatory stress, and may also involve, in the elderly, a low-grade systemic inflammatory response or insulin resistance. However, none of these inflammatory conditions match the definition of cachexia (Muscaritoli et al., 2010). Ageing is characterised by quantitative and qualitative modifications of the immune system. This phenomenon, known as '**immunosenescence**', is accompanied by cytokine dysregulation, which is an increase of pro-inflammatory cytokines and reduction of anti-inflammatory cytokines, leading to a chronic low-grade inflammatory state (Miller, 1996).

Sarcopenic obesity

An age-dependent decline in skeletal muscle mass, strength and endurance during the ageing process is a physiological development, but several factors may exacerbate this process, leading to the threatening state of sarcopenia, frailty and, eventually, higher mortality rates. Obesity appears to be such a promoting factor and has been linked in several studies to sarcopenia. The reason for this causal association remains poorly understood (Kob et al., 2015).

Obesity is characterised by endocrine changes and visceral fat deposits produce more pro-inflammatory adipokines leading to a low-grade inflammatory state (Schrager et al., 2007). Loss of lean body mass, reduced immune function, cognitive decline, accelerated atherosclerosis and insulin resistance are the consequences of this low-grade inflammatory state (e.g. Zamboni et al., 2008).

Sarcopenic obesity (SO) in conditions such as malignancy, rheumatoid arthritis and ageing, lean body mass is lost while fat mass may be preserved or even increased (Prado et al., 2008). The relationship between age-related reduction of muscle mass and strength is often independent of body mass. SO is described as a syndrome characterised by the rise of body fat mass in parallel with excessive low muscle mass, with underlying elements such as endocrine, inflammatory and lifestyle disruptions

(Wannamethee and Atkins, 2015; Zamboni et al., 2008). SO is highly correlated with metabolism-related disease, chronic disease and functional disabilities, and has been described as 'thin outside, fat inside' or 'TOFI' (Stenholm et al., 2008). Sarcopenic obesity appears to be linked with the up-regulation of TNF-α, interleukin (IL)-6, leptin and myostatin, and the down-regulation of adiponectin and IL-15. Multiple combined exercise and mild caloric restriction markedly attenuate the symptoms of sarcopenic obesity. Intriguingly, the inhibition of myostatin induced by gene manipulation or neutralising antibody ameliorates sarcopenic obesity via increased skeletal muscle mass and improved glucose homeostasis (Sakuma and Yamaguchi, 2013).

Finally, a major gap in knowledge is the lack of data for minority ethnic groups. Ethnic differences in the prevalence or incidence of sarcopenia, its pathogenesis and its consequences are largely unknown. Most epidemiologic studies of impairment, disability, falls and other risk factors for sarcopenia have been of white, middle-class, elderly cohorts, and few studies have included ethnic minorities (Morley et al., 2001).

References

Ahmed T, Haboubi N. (2010). Assessment and management of nutrition in older people and its importance to health. *Clin Interv Aging.* August 9; 5: 207–16.

Annweiler C, Beauchet O, Berrut G, Fantino B, Bonnefoy M, Herrmann FR, Schott MA et al. (2009). Is there an association between serum 25-hydroxyvitamin D concentration and muscle strength among older women? Results from baseline assessment of the EPIDOS study. *J. Nutr. Health Aging.* 13: 90–5.

Bauer JM, Kaiser MJ, Sieber CC. (2008). Sarcopenia in nursing home residents. *J Am Med Dir Assoc.* October; 9(8): 545–51. doi:10.1016/j.jamda.2008.04.010.

Baumgartner RN, Waters LW. (2006). Sarcopenia and sarcopenic-obesity. In: Pathy MS, Sinclair AJ, Morley JE (eds), *Principles and practice of geriatric medicine.* Chichester: John Wiley & Sons, pp. 909–33.

Baumgartner R, Koehler KM, Gallagher D, Romero L, Heymsfield SB, Ross RR, Garry PJ, Lindeman RD. (1998). Epidemiology of sarcopenia among the elderly in New Mexico. *Am. J. Epidemiol.* 147: 755–63.

Beaudart C, McCloskey E, Bruyère O, Cesari M, Rolland Y, Rizzoli R, Araujo de Carvalho I, Amuthavalli Thiyagarajan J, Bautmans I, Bertière MC, Brandi ML, Al-Daghri NM, Burlet N, Cavalier E, Cerreta F, Cherubini A, Fielding R, Gielen E, Landi F, Petermans J, Reginster JY, Visser M, Kanis J, Cooper C. (2016). Sarcopenia in daily practice: assessment and management. *BMC Geriatr.* October 5; 16(1): 170.

Bernabei R, Mariotti L, Bordes P, Roubenoff R. (2017). The 'Sarcopenia and Physical fRailty IN older people: multi-componenT Treatment strategies' (SPRINTT) project: advancing the care of physically frail and sarcopenic older people. *Aging Clin Exp Res.* February; 29(1): 1–2. doi:10.1007/s40520-016-0707-2. Epub 2017 January 31.

Bischoff-Ferrari HA, Dawson-Hughes B, Staehelin HB, Orav JE, Stuck AE, Theiler R et al. (2009). Fall prevention with supplemental and active forms of vitamin D: a meta-analysis of randomised controlled trials. *BMJ.* 339: b3692.

Bischoff-Ferrari HA, Dawson-Hughes B, Willett WC, Staehelin HB, Bazemore MG, Zee RY, Wong JB. (2004). Effect of Vitamin D on falls: a meta-analysis. *JAMA.* April 28; 291(16): 1999-2006.

Bolland MJ, Bacon CJ, Horne AM, Mason BH, Ruth W Ames RW, Wang TKM *et al.* (2010). Vitamin D insufficiency and health outcomes over 5 y in older women. *J Am Geriatr Soc.* 25: 82–9.

Bowen TS, Schuler G, Adams V. (2015). Skeletal muscle wasting in cachexia and sarcopenia: molecular pathophysiology and impact of exercise training. *Cachexia Sarcopenia Muscle.* September; 6(3): 197–207. doi:10.1002/jcsm.12043. Epub 2015 June 3.

Buckinx F, Landi F, Cesari M, Fielding RA, Visser M, Engelke K, Maggi S, Dennison E, Al-Daghri NM, Allepaerts S, Bauer J, Bautmans I, Brandi ML, Bruyère O, Cederholm T, Cerreta F, Cherubini A, Cooper C, Cruz-Jentoft A, McCloskey E, Dawson-Hughes B, Kaufman JM, Laslop A, Petermans J, Reginster JY, Rizzoli R, Robinson S, Rolland Y, Rueda R, Vellas B, Kanis JA. (2018). Pitfalls in the measurement of muscle mass: a need for a reference standard. *J Cachexia Sarcopenia Muscle.* January 19. doi:10.1002/jcsm.12268. [Epub ahead of print].

Buford TW, Anton SD, Judge AR, Marzetti E, Wohlgemuth SE, Carter CS, Leeuwenburgh C. *et al.* (2010). Models of accelerated sarcopenia: critical pieces for solving the puzzle of age-related muscle atrophy. *Ageing Res Rev.* 9: 369–83.

Calvani R, Marini F, Cesari M, Tosato M, Anker SD, von Haehling S, Miller RR, Bernabei R, Landi F, Marzetti E; SPRINTT consortium. (2015). Biomarkers for physical frailty and sarcopenia: state of the science and future developments. *J Cachexia Sarcopenia Muscle.* December; 6(4): 278–86. doi:10.1002/jcsm.12051. Epub 2015 July 7.

Calvani R, Miccheli A, Landi F, Bossola M, Cesari M, Leeuwenburgh C, Sieber CC, Bernabei R, Marzetti E. (2013). Current nutritional recommendations and novel dietary strategies to manage sarcopenia. *J Frailty Aging.* 2(1): 38–53.

Calvani R, Picca A, Marini F, Biancolillo A, Cesari M, Pesce V, Lezza AMS, Bossola M, Leeuwenburgh C, Bernabei R, Landi F, Marzetti E. (2018). The 'BIOmarkers associated with Sarcopenia and PHysical frailty in EldeRly pErsons' (BIOSPHERE) study: rationale, design and methods. *Eur J Intern Med.* May 10. pii: S0953-6205(18)30178-X. doi:10.1016/j.ejim.2018.05.001. [Epub ahead of print].

Cao Dinh H, Beyer I, Mets T, Onyema OO, Njemini R, Renmans W, De Waele M, Jochmans K, Vander Meeren S, Bautmans I. (2017). Effects of physical exercise on markers of cellular immunosenescence: a systematic review. *Calcif Tissue Int.* February; 100(2): 193–215. doi:10.1007/s00223-016-0212-9. Epub 2016 November 19.

Cartee GD, Hepple RT, Bamman MM, Zierath JR. (2016). Exercise promotes healthy aging of skeletal muscle. *Cell Metabolism.* 23(6): 1034–47. doi:10.1016/j.cmet.2016.05.007.

Cawthon PM, Peters KW, Shardell MD, McLean RR, Dam TT, Kenny AM, Fragala MS, Harris TB, Kiel DP, Guralnik JM, Ferrucci L, Kritchevsky SB, Vassileva MT, Studenski SA, Alley DE. (2014). Cutpoints for low appendicular lean mass that identify older adults with clinically significant weakness. *J Gerontol A Biol Sci Med Sci.* 69(5): 567–75.

Ceglia L, Chiu GR, Harris SS, Araujo AB. (2011). Serum 25-hydroxyvitamin D concentration and physical function in adult men. *Clin Endocrinol (Oxf).* 74: 370–6.

Chang SS, Weiss CO, Xue QL, Fried LP. (2012). Association between inflammatory-related disease burden and frailty: results from the Women's Health and Aging Studies (WHAS) I and II. *Arch Gerontol Geriatr.* January–February; 54(1): 9–15. doi:10.1016/j.archger.2011.05.020. Epub 2011 July 16.

Cheek DB. (1985). The control of cell mass and replication: the DNA unita personal 20-year study. *Early Hum Dev.* 12: 211–39.

Chumlea WC, Cesari M, Evans WJ, Ferrucci L, Fielding RA, Pahor M, Studenski S, Vellas B; International Working Group on Sarcopenia Task Force Members. (2011). Sarcopenia: designing phase IIB trials. *J Nutr Health Aging.* June; 15(6): 450–5.

Coto-Montes A, Boga JA, Tan DX, Reiter RJ. (2016). Melatonin as a potential agent in the treatment of sarcopenia. *Int J Mol Sci*. October 24; 17(10). pii: E1771.

Crews DE. (2007). Senescence, aging, and disease. *J Physiol Anthropol*. May; 26(3): 365–72.

Cruz-Jentoft AJ, Michel J-P. (2013). Sarcopenia: a useful paradigm for physical frailty. *Eur Geriatr Med*. 4: 102–5.

Cruz-Jentoft AJ, Baeyens JP, Bauer JM, Boirie Y, Cederholm T, Landi F *et al*. (2010). Sarcopenia: European consensus on definition and diagnosis: Report of the European Working Group on Sarcopenia in Older People. *Age Ageing*. 39: 412–23.

Cruz-Jentoft AJ, Landi F, Schneider SM, Zuniga C, Arai H, Boirie Y, Chen L-K, Fielding RA, Martin FC, Michel J-P, Sieber C, Stout JR, Studenski SA, Vellas B, Woo J, Zamboni M, Cederholm T. (2014). Prevalence of and interventions for sarcopenia in ageing adults: a systematic review. Report of the International Sarcopenia Initiative (EWGSOP and IWGS). *Age Ageing*. 43: 748–59. doi:10.1093/ageing/afu115.

Dardevet D, Savary-Auzeloux I, Remond D, Mosoni L, Marzetti E, Buford TW, Bernabei R. *et al*. (2012). Commentaries on viewpoint: muscle atrophy is not always sarcopenia. *J Appl Physiol*. (1985) 113: 680–4.

DeFronzo RA, Tripathy D. (2009). Skeletal muscle insulin resistance is the primary defect in type 2 diabetes. *Diabetes Care*. November; 32(Suppl. 2): S157–63. doi:10.2337/dc09-S302.

De Martinis M, Franceschi C, Monti D, Ginaldi L. (2006). Inflammation markers predicting frailty and mortality in the elderly. *Exp Mol Pathol*. June; 80(3): 219–27. Epub 2006 February 7.

Del Signore S, Roubenoff R. (2017). Physical frailty and sarcopenia (PF&S): a point of view from the industry. *Aging Clin Exp Res*. February; 29(1): 69–74. doi:10.1007/s40520-016-0710-7. Epub 2017 February 3.

Dhillon RJ, Hasni S. (2017). Pathogenesis and Management of Sarcopenia. *Clin Geriatr Med*. February; 33(1): 17–26. doi:10.1016/j.cger.2016.08.002.

Di Monaco M, Vallero F, Di Monaco R, Tappero R. (2011). Prevalence of sarcopenia and its association with osteoporosis in 313 older women following a hip fracture. *Arch Gerontol Geriatr*. January–February; 52(1): 71–4. doi:10.1016/j.archger.2010.02.002. Epub 2010 Mar 5.

Drummond MJ, Rasmussen BB. (2008). Leucine-enriched nutrients and the regulation of mammalian target of rapamycin signalling and human skeletal muscle protein synthesis. *Curr Opin Clin Nutr Metab Care*. May; 11(3): 222–6. doi:10.1097/MCO.0b013e3282fa17fb.

Dupont-Versteegden EE. (2005). Apoptosis in muscle atrophy: relevance to sarcopenia. *Exp Gerontol*. June; 40(6): 473–81.

Egan B, Zierath JR. (2013). Exercise metabolism and the molecular regulation of skeletal muscle adaptation. *Cell Metabolism*. 17(2): 162–84.

Fielding RA, Vellas B, Evans WJ, Bhasin S, Morley JE, Newman AB *et al*. (2011). Sarcopenia: an undiagnosed condition in older adults. Current consensus definition: Prevalence, etiology, and consequences. International working group on sarcopenia. *J Am Med Dir Assoc*. 12: 249–56.

Fougère B, Sourdet S, Lilamand M, Tabue-Teguod M, Teysseyre B, Dupuy C, Vellas B, Rolland Y, Nourhashemi F, van Kan GA. (2018). Untangling the overlap between frailty and low lean mass: data from Toulouse frailty day hospital. *Arch Gerontol Geriatr*. March–April; 75: 209–13. doi:10.1016/j.archger.2017.12.013. Epub 2017 December 29.

Fragala MS, Dam TT, Barber V, Judge JO, Studenski SA, Cawthon PM, McLean RR, Harris TB, Ferrucci L, Guralnik JM, Kiel DP, Kritchevsky SB, Shardell MD, Vassileva MT, Kenny AM. (2015). Strength and function response to clinical interventions of older women categorized by weakness and low lean mass using classifications from the

Foundation for the National Institute of Health sarcopenia project. *J Gerontol A Biol Sci Med Sci.* February; 70(2): 202–9. doi:10.1093/gerona/glu110. Epub 2014 August 18.

Frontera WLJ. (2005). Assessment of human muscle function. In: De Lisa J, Gans BM, Walsh NE (eds), *Physical medicine and rehabilitation*, 1st edn. Philadelphia, PA: Lippincott Williams & Wilkins, pp. 139–54.

Frost RA, Nystrom GJ, Lang CH. (2003). Tumor necrosis factor-alpha decreases insulin-like growth factor-I messenger ribonucleic acid expression in C2C12 myoblasts via a Jun N-terminal kinase pathway. *Endocrinology.* May; 144(5): 1770–9.

Gillespie LD, Robertson MC, Gillespie WJ, Lamb SE, Gates S, Cumming RG, Rowe BH. (2009). Interventions for preventing falls in older people living in the community. *Cochrane Database Syst Rev.* CD007146.

Gleeson M, Walsh NP. (2012). The BASES expert statement on exercise, immunity, and infection. *J Sports Sci.* 30: 321–4. doi:10.1080/02640414.2011.627371.

Guralnik JM, Simonsick EM, Ferrucci L, Glynn RJ, Berkman LF, Blazer DG, Scherr PA, Wallace RB. (1994). A short physical performance battery assessing lower extremity function: association with self-reported disability and prediction of mortality and nursing home admission. *J Gerontol.* March; 49(2): M85–94.

Harada H, Kai H, Shibata R, Niiyama H, Nishiyama Y, Murohara T, Yoshida N, Katoh A, Ikeda H. (2017). New diagnostic index for sarcopenia in patients with cardiovascular diseases. *PLoS One.* May 18; 12(5): e0178123. doi:10.1371/journal.pone.0178123. eCollection 2017.

Heymsfield SB, Gonzalez MC, Lu J, Jia G, Zheng J. (2015). Skeletal muscle mass and quality: evolution of modern measurement concepts in the context of sarcopenia. *Proc Nutr Soc.* November; 74(4): 355–66. doi:10.1017/S0029665115000129. Epub 2015 April 8.

Houston DK, Nicklas BJ, Ding J, Harris TB, Tylavsky FA, Newman AB *et al.* (2008). Dietary protein intake is associated with lean mass change in older, community-dwelling adults: the Health, Aging, and Body Composition (Health ABC) Study. *Am J Clin Nutr.* 87: 150–5.

Kalinkovich A, Livshits G. (2015). Sarcopenia: the search for emerging biomarkers. *Ageing Res Rev.* 22: 58–71.

Kamel HK. (2003). Sarcopenia and aging. *Nutr Rev.* 61: 157–67.

Kashani K, Sarvottam K, Pereira NL, Barreto EF, Kennedy CC. (2017). The Sarcopenia Index: a novel measure of muscle mass in lung transplant candidates. *Clin Transplant.* December 23. doi:10.1111/ctr.13182. [Epub ahead of print].

Keevil VL, Romero-Ortuno R. (2015). Ageing well: a review of sarcopenia and frailty. *Proceedings of the Nutrition Society* (Cambridge). November; 74(4): 337–47.

Kob R, Bollheimer LC, Bertsch T, Fellner C, Djukic M, Sieber CC, Fischer BE. (2015). Sarcopenic obesity: molecular clues to a better understanding of its pathogenesis? *Biogerontology.* February; 16(1): 15–29. doi:10.1007/s10522-014-9539-7. Epub 2014 November 7.

Landi F, Cesari M, Calvani R, Cherubini A, Di Bari M, Bejuit R, Mshid J, Andrieu S, Sinclair AJ, Sieber CC, Vellas B, Topinkova E, Strandberg T, Rodriguez-Manas L, Lattanzio F, Pahor M, Roubenoff R, Cruz-Jentoft AJ, Bernabei R, Marzetti E; SPRINTT Consortium. (2017). The 'Sarcopenia and Physical fRailty IN older people: multicomponenT Treatment strategies' (SPRINTT) randomized controlled trial: design and methods. *Aging Clin Exp Res.* February; 29(1): 89–100. doi:10.1007/s40520-016-0715-2. Epub 2017 January 31.

Laosa O, Alonso C, Castro M, Rodriguez-Manas L. (2014). Pharmaceutical interventions for frailty and sarcopenia. *Curr Pharm Des.* 20: 3068–82.

Lardiés-Sánchez B, Sanz-París A, Pérez-Nogueras J, Serrano-Oliver A, Torres-Anoro ME, Cruz-Jentoft AJ. (2017). Influence of nutritional status in the diagnosis of sarcopenia in nursing home residents. *Nutrition.* September; 41: 51–7. doi:10.1016/j.nut.2017.03.002. Epub 2017 April 7.

LeBrasseur NK, Tchkonia T, Kirkland JL. (2015). Cellular senescence and the biology of aging, disease, and frailty. *Nestle Nutr Inst Workshop Ser.* 83: 11–18. doi:10.1159/000382054. Epub 2015 October 20.

Leslie WD, Majumdar SR, Lix LM, Johansson H, Oden A, McCloskey E, Kanis JA; Manitoba Bone Density Program. (2012). High fracture probability with FRAX usually indicates densitometric osteoporosis: implications for clinical practice. *Osteoporos Int.* 23: 391–7.

Levine JA, Abboud L, Barry M, Reed JE, Sheedy PF, Jensen MD. (2000). Measuring leg muscle and fat mass in humans: comparison of CT and dual energy X-ray absorptiometry. *J Appl Physiol.* 88: 452–6.

Liccini A, Malmstrom TK. (2016). Frailty and sarcopenia as predictors of adverse health outcomes in persons with diabetes mellitus. *J Am Med Dir Assoc.* September 1; 17(9): 846–51. doi:10.1016/j.jamda.2016.07.007.

Liu CJ, Latham NK. (2009). Progressive resistance strength training for improving physical function in older adults. *Cochrane Database Syst Rev.* 3: CD002759.

Liu CK, Lyass A, Larson MG, Massaro JM, Wang N, D'Agostino Sr RB, Benjamin EJ, Murabito JM. (2016). Biomarkers of oxidative stress are associated with frailty: the Framingham Offspring Study. *Age* (Dordr). 38: 1.

Malmstrom TK, Morley JE. (2013). Sarcopenia: the target population. *J Frailty Aging.* 2: 55–6.

Martone AM, Marzetti E, Calvani R, Picca A, Tosato M, Santoro L, Di Giorgio A, Nesci A, Sisto A, Santoliquido A, Landi F. (2017). Exercise and protein intake: a synergistic approach against sarcopenia. *Biomed Res Int.* 2017: 2672435. doi:10.1155/2017/2672435. Epub 2017 March 21.

Marzetti E, Calvani R, Cesari M, Tosato M, Cherubini A, Di Bari M, Pahor M, Savera G, Collamati A, D'Angelo E, Bernabei R, Landi F. (2016). Operationalization of the physical frailty and sarcopenia syndrome: rationale and clinical implementation. *Transl Med UniSa.* January 31; 13: 29–32. eCollection 2015 December.

Marzetti E, Calvani R, Tosato M, Cesari M, Di Bari M, Cherubini A, Collamati A, D'Angelo E, Pahor M, Bernabei R, Landi F; SPRINTT Consortium. (2017). Sarcopenia: an overview. *Aging Clin Exp Res.* February; 29(1): 11–17. doi:10.1007/s40520-016-0704-5. Epub 2017 February 2. Review.

McLean RR, Kiel DP. (2015). Developing consensus criteria for sarcopenia: an update. *J Bone Miner Res.* April; 30(4): 588–92. doi:10.1002/jbmr.2492.

Michaud M, Balardy L, Moulis G, Gaudin C, Peyrot C, Vellas B, Cesari M, Nourhashemi F. (2013). Proinflammatory cytokines, aging, and age-related diseases. *J Am Med Dir Assoc.* December; 14(12): 877–82. doi:10.1016/j.jamda.2013.05.009. Epub 2013 June 20.

Michel JP, Cruz-Jentoft AJ, Cederholm T. (2015). Frailty, exercise and nutrition. *Clin Geriatr Med.* August; 31(3): 375–87. doi:10.1016/j.cger.2015.04.006. Epub 2015 May 13.

Miller RA. (1996). The aging immune system: primer and prospectus. *Science.* 273: 70–4.

Milne AC, Potter J, Vivanti A, Avenell A. (2009). Protein and energy supplementation in elderly people at risk from malnutrition. *Cochrane Database Syst Rev.* April 15; 2: CD003288. doi:10.1002/14651858.CD003288.pub3.

Morley JE. (2008). Sarcopenia: diagnosis and treatment. *J Nutr Health Aging.* 12: 452–6.

Morley JE. (2016). Frailty and sarcopenia in elderly. *Wien Klin Wochenschr.* December; 128(Suppl. 7): 439–45. Epub 2016 September 26.

Morley JE, Malmstrom TK. (2013). Frailty, sarcopenia, and hormones. *Endocrinol Metab Clin North Am.* June; 42(2): 391–405. doi:10.1016/j.ecl.2013.02.006.

Morley JE, Abbatecola AM, Argiles JM, Baracos V, Bauer J, Bhasin S, Cederholm T, Coats AJ, Cummings SR, Evans WJ, Fearon K, Ferrucci L, Fielding RA, Guralnik JM, Harris TB, Inui A, Kalantar-Zadeh K, Kirwan BA, Mantovani G, Muscaritoli M, Newman AB, Rossi-Fanelli F, Rosano GM, Roubenoff R, Schambelan M, Sokol GH, Storer TW, Vellas B, von Haehling S, Yeh SS, Anker SD; Society on Sarcopenia, Cachexia and Wasting Disorders Trialist Workshop. (2011). Sarcopenia with limited mobility: an international consensus. *J Am Med Dir Assoc.* July; 12(6): 403–9. doi:10.1016/j.jamda.2011.04.014.

Morley JE, Baumgartner RN, Roubenoff R, Mayer J, Nair KS. (2001). Sarcopenia. *J Lab Clin Med.* April; 137(4): 231–43.

Muscaritoli M, Anker SD, Argilés J, Aversa Z, Bauer JM, Biolo G, Boirie Y, Bosaeus I, Cederholm T, Costelli P, Fearon KC, Laviano A, Maggio M, Rossi Fanelli F, Schneider SM, Schols A, Sieber CC. (2010). Consensus definition of sarcopenia, cachexia and pre-cachexia: joint document elaborated by Special Interest Groups (SIG) 'cachexia-anorexia in chronic wasting diseases' and 'nutrition in geriatrics'. *Clin Nutr.* April; 29(2): 154–9. doi:10.1016/j.clnu.2009.12.004. Epub 2010 January 8.

Navratil M, Terman A, Arriaga EA. (2008). Giant mitochondria do not fuse and exchange their contents with normal mitochondria. *Exp Cell Res.* 314: 164–72.

Newman AB, Lee JS, Visser M, Goodpaster BH, Kritchevsky SB, Tylavsky FA, Nevitt M, Harris TB. (2005). Weight change and the conservation of lean mass in old age: the health, aging and body composition study. *Am J Clin Nutr.* 82: 872–8.

Nielsen HB. (2003). Lymphocyte responses to maximal exercise. *Sports Med.* 33(11): 853–67.

Pahor M, Guralnik JM, Ambrosius WT, Blair S, Bonds DE, Church TS, Espeland MA, Fielding RA, Gill TM, Groessl EJ, King AC, Kritchevsky SB, Manini TM, McDermott MM, Miller ME, Newman AB, Rejeski WJ, Sink KM, Williamson JD; LIFE study investigators (2014) Effect of structured physical activity on prevention of major mobility disability in older adults: the LIFE study randomized clinical trial. *JAMA.* 311: 2387–96. doi:10.1001/jama.2014.5616.

Pannérec A, Springer M, Migliavacca E, Ireland A, Piasecki M, Karaz S, Jacot G, Métairon S, Danenberg E, Raymond F, Descombes P, McPhee JS, Feige JN. (2016). A robust neuromuscular system protects rat and human skeletal muscle from sarcopenia. *Aging* (Albany, NY). Apr; 8(4): 712–29. doi:10.18632/aging.100926.

Park SW, Goodpaster BH, Strotmeyer ES, Kuller LH, Broudeau R, Kammerer C, de Rekeneire N, Harris TB, Schwartz AV, Tylavsky FA, Cho YW, Newman AB; Health, Aging, and Body Composition Study. (2007). Accelerated loss of skeletal muscle strength in older adults with type 2 diabetes: the health, aging, and body composition study. *Diabetes Care.* 30: 1507–12.

Park SW, Goodpaster BH, Lee JS, Kuller LH, Boudreau R, de Rekeneire N, Harris TB, Kritchevsky S, Tylavsky FA, Nevitt M, Cho YW, Newman AB; Health, Aging, and Body Composition Study. (2009). Excessive loss of skeletal muscle mass in older adults with type 2 diabetes. *Diabetes Care.* 32: 1993–7. [PMC free article].

Pattison JS, Folk LC, Madsen RW, Childs TE, Booth FW. (2003). Transcriptional profiling identifies extensive downregulation of extracellular matrix gene expression in sarcopenic rat soleus muscle. *Physiol Genomics.* 15(1): 34–43.

Pedersen BK, Toft AD. (2000). Effects of exercise on lymphocyte and cytokines. *Br J Sports Med.* 34: 246–251.

Pourhassan M, Norman K, Müller MJ, Dziewas R, Wirth R. (2018). Impact of sarcopenia on one-year mortality among older hospitalized patients with impaired mobility. *J Frailty Aging*. 7(1): 40–6. doi:10.14283/jfa.2017.35.

Prado CM, Lieffers JR, McCargar LJ, Reiman T, Sawyer MB, Martin L, Baracos VE. (2008). Prevalence and clinical implications of sarcopenic obesity in patients with solid tumours of the respiratory and gastrointestinal tracts: a population-based study. *Lancet Oncol*. 9: 629–35.

Puthucheary ZA, Rawal J, McPhail M, Connolly B, Ratnayake G, Chan P, Hopkinson NS, Phadke R, Dew T, Sidhu PS, Velloso C, Seymour J, Agley CC, Selby A, Limb M, Edwards LM, Smith K, Rowlerson A, Rennie MJ, Moxham J, Harridge SD, Hart N, Montgomery HE. (2013). Acute skeletal muscle wasting in critical illness. *JAMA*. October 16; 310(15): 1591–600.

Reginster JY, Cooper C, Rizzoli R, Kanis JA, Appelboom G, Bautmans I, Bischo-Ferrari HA, Boers M, Brandi ML, Bruyère O, Cherubini A, Flamion B, Fielding RA, Gasparik AI, Van Loon L, McCloskey E, Mitlak BH, Pilotto A, Reiter-Niesert S, Rolland Y, Tsouderos Y, Visser M, Cruz-Jentoft AJ. (2016). Recommendations for the conduct of clinical trials for drugs to treat or prevent sarcopenia. *Aging Clin Exp Res*. 28: 47–58.

Reijnierse EM, Trappenburg MC, Blauw GJ, Verlaan S, de van der Schueren MA, Meskers CG, Maier AB. (2016). Common ground? The concordance of sarcopenia and frailty definitions. *J Am Med Dir Assoc*. April 1; 17(4): 371.e7–12. doi:10.1016/j.jamda.2016.01.013. Epub 2016 February 24.

Rolland Y, Dupuy C, Abellan Van Kan G, Cesari M, Vellas B, Faruch M, Dray C, de Souto Barreto P. (2017). Sarcopenia screened by the SARC-F Questionnaire and physical performances of elderly women: a cross-sectional study. *J Am Med Dir Assoc*. October 1; 18(10): 848–52. doi:10.1016/j.jamda.2017.05.010. Epub 2017 June 16.

Romera L, Orfila F, Segura JM, Ramirez A, Möller M, Fabra ML, Lancho S, Bastida N, Foz G, Fabregat MA, Martí N, Cullell M, Martinez D, Giné M, Bistuer A, Cendrós P, Pérez E. (2014). Effectiveness of a primary care based multifactorial intervention to improve frailty parameters in the elderly: a randomised clinical trial: rationale and study design. *BMC Geriatr*. November 27; 14: 125. doi:10.1186/1471-2318-14-125.

Rosenberg IH. (1989). Summary comments. *Am J Clin Nutr*. 50: 1231, 1232–3.

Sakuma K, Yamaguchi A. (2013). Sarcopenic obesity and endocrinal adaptation with age. *Int J Endocrinol*. 2013: 204164. doi:10.1155/2013/204164. Epub 2013 April 11.

Sayer AA. (2014). Sarcopenia the new geriatric giant: time to translate research findings into clinical practice. *Age Ageing*. November; 43(6): 736–7. doi:10.1093/ageing/afu118. Epub 2014 September 16.

Schaap LA, Pluijm SM, Deeg DJ, Visser M. (2006). Inflammatory markers and loss of muscle mass (sarcopenia) and strength. *Am J Med*. June; 119(6): 526.e9–17.

Schrager MA, Metter EJ, Simonsick E, Ble A, Bandinelli S, Lauretani F, Ferrucci L (2007). Sarcopenic obesity and inflammation in the InCHIANTI study. *J Appl Physiol*. 102: 919–25.

Scott D, Hayes A, Sanders KM, Aitken D, Ebeling PR, Jones G. (2014). Operational definitions of sarcopenia and their associations with 5-year changes in falls risk in community-dwelling middle-aged and older adults. *Osteoporosis International*. 25(1): 187–93.

Shaw SC, Dennison EM, Cooper C. (2017). Epidemiology of sarcopenia: determinants throughout the lifecourse. *Calcif Tissue Int*. September; 101(3): 229–47. doi:10.1007/s00223-017-0277-0. Epub 2017 April 18.

Shaw AC, Joshi S, Greenwood H, Panda A, Lord JM. (2010). Aging of the innate immune system. *Curr Opin Immunol*. 22: 507–13.

Sinclair AJ, Abdelhafiz AH, Rodríguez-Mañas L. (2017). Frailty and sarcopenia: newly emerging and high impact complications of diabetes. *J Diabetes Complications*. September; 31(9): 1465–73. doi:10.1016/j.jdiacomp. Epub 2017 May 12.

Singh T, Newman AB. (2011). Inflammatory markers in population studies of aging. *Ageing Res Rev.* July; 10(3): 319–29. doi:10.1016/j.arr.2010.11.002. Epub 2010 December 8.

Springer J, Springer JI, Anker SD. (2017). Muscle wasting and sarcopenia in heart failure and beyond: update 2017. *ESC Heart Fail.* November; 4(4): 492–8. doi:10.1002/ehf2.12237.

Stenholm S, Harris TB, Rantanen T, Visser M, Kritchevsky SB, Ferrucci L. (2008). Sarcopenic obesity: definition, cause and consequences. *Curr Opin Clin Nutr Metab Care.* November; 11(6): 693–700. doi:10.1097/MCO.0b013e328312c37d.

Stockton KA, Mengersen K, Paratz JD, Kandiah D, Bennell KL. (2011). Effect of vitamin D supplementation on muscle strength: a systematic review and meta-analysis. *Osteoporos Int.* 22: 859–71.

Studenski SA, Peters KW, Alley DE, Cawthon PM, McLean RR, Harris TB *et al.* (2014). The FNIH sarcopenia project: rationale, study description, conference recommendations, and final estimates. *J Gerontol A Biol Sci Med Sci.* 69: 547–58.

Toth MJ, Ades PA, Tischler MD, Tracy RP, LeWinter MM. (2006). Immune activation is associated with reduced skeletal muscle mass and physical function in chronic heart failure. *Int J Cardiol.* 109: 179–87. doi:10.1016/j. ijcard.2005.06.006.

Turner JE. (2016). Is immunosenescence influenced by our lifetime 'dose' of exercise? *Biogerontology.* June; 17(3): 581–602. doi:10.1007/s10522-016-9642-z. Epub 2016 March 29.

Van Epps P, Oswald D, Higgins PA, Hornick TR, Aung H, Banks RE, Wilson BM, Burant C, Graventstein S, Canaday DH. (2016). Frailty has a stronger association with inflammation than age in older veterans. *Immun Ageing.* October 19; 13: 27. eCollection 2016.

Vanderwoude MF, Alish CJ, Sauer AC, Hegazi RA. (2012). Malnutrition-sarcopenia syndrome: is this the future of nutrition screening and assessment for older adults? *J Aging Res.* 2012; 2012: 651570. Epub 2012 September 13.

Vasilaki A, Mansouri A, Remmen H., van der Meulen JH, Larkin L, Richardson AG *et al.* (2006). Free radical generation by skeletal muscle of adult and old mice: effect of contractile activity. *Aging Cell.* 5: 109–17.

Visser M, Pahor M, Taaffe DR, Goodpaster BH, Simonsick EM, Newman AB, Nevitt M, Harris TB. (2002). Relationship of interleukin-6 and tumor necrosis factor alpha with muscle mass and muscle strength in elderly men and women: the Health ABC Study. *J Gerontol A Biol Sci Med Sci.* 57: M326–32.

von Haehling S, Morley JE, Anker SD. (2010). An overview of sarcopenia: facts and numbers on prevalence and clinical impact. *J Cachexia Sarcopenia Muscle.* December; 1(2): 129–33. Epub 2010 December 17.

Wannamethee SG, Atkins JL. (2015). Muscle loss and obesity: the health implications of sarcopenia and sarcopenic obesity. *Proceedings of the Nutrition Society.* 74(4): 405–12. http://dx.doi.org/10.1017/S002966511500169X.

Wilson D, Jackson T, Sapey E, Lord JM. (2017). Frailty and sarcopenia: the potential role of an aged immune system. *Ageing Res Rev.* July; 36: 1–10. doi:10.1016/j.arr.2017.01.006. Epub 2017 February 20.

Yu SC, Khow KS, Jadczak AD, Visvanathan R. (2016). Clinical screening tools for sarcopenia and its management. *Curr Gerontol Geriatr Res.* 2016:5978523. doi:10.1155/2016/5978523. Epub 2016 February 4.

Zamboni M, Mazzali G, Fantin F, Rossi A, Di Francesco V. (2008). Sarcopenicobesity: a new category of obesity in the elderly. *Nutr Metab Cardiovasc Dis.*18: 388–95.

Zoico E, Corzato F, Bambace C, Rossi AP, Micciolo R, Cinti S, Harris TB, Zambonia M. (2013). Myosteatosis and myofibrosis: relationship with aging, inflammation and insulin resistance. *Arch Gerontol Geriatrics.* 57(3): 411–16.

6

INTERVENTIONS IN FRAILTY CARE AND ENHANCING INDEPENDENCE

Aim

After a person has been identified as being frail, it makes sense to offer practical ways of improving the frailty and, at the very least, to prevent the frailty from getting worse. The aims of care and support should be to encourage health, wellbeing and independence, and to discourage disability, dependence and illness. I wish to evaluate critically a number of key interventions in this chapter as examples.

Introduction

If recognised early, there are interventions to improve independence and quality of life for people living with frailty. 'Interventions' very much fit into the biomedical model of viewing frailty, with an intervention actively done to a patient who is frail to improve outcomes in health and wellbeing. As such, interventions should utilise a goal-orientated rather than a disease-focused approach. An alternative view is that a healthy environment should be promoted to build up assets and resilience for all persons living with frailty. At one extreme, it might be that people who are frail are repelled by the world around them when the environment wants to 'erase' frailty (see a challenging sociological discourse by Joanna Latimer[1]).

It seems that, while the literature contains a large number of interventions for frail older adults, there are few studies specifically addressing frailty using validated scales or measurements of frailty as initial measures and primary outcome, with a general older population (Apóstolo *et al.*, 2018). Interventions which are multi-dimensional and home-based tend to target either broader or frailer populations, have had mixed success so far, and can lack clarity as to their effective '**active ingredients**' (Frost *et al.*, 2017). It is important to work with people living with frailty and others to co-produce a care and support plan that balances interventions with the needs and wishes of the person. It is becoming increasingly recognised that frailty requires an integrated and interdisciplinary response through social co-production across traditional boundaries and 'silos' (Gwyther *et al.*, 2018). This would require a culture shift in care with redeployment of existing resources to deliver frailty management and intervention services.

Hospitalisations can indeed be a problem as well as a solution.

A tension remains between interventions which are thought of as at a **population level**, where clearly, because of the nature of the complexity of frailty, interventions need to be offered in a holistic integrated **person-centred** way. For example, it was recently noted that 'It is tempting to think that interventions should be personalized and a holistic approach taken. Most certainly, they should be multifaceted e.g. reduction of polypharmacy, encouraging engagement in social life, and vision correction among others' (McGuigan *et al.*, 207, p. 154). On the other hand, it is argued that

> We need a culture in which we do not see 'sarcopenia' or 'frailty' as distinct entities such as rheumatoid arthritis, but as the end of distribution curves which need a population based approach where the knowledge and expertise of the professions such as medicine, physiotherapy, nursing and occupational therapy being mobilised digitally and delivered directly.
>
> *(Gray and Butler, 2017, p. 259)*

From a plethora of stakeholder/public perspectives, new frailty prevention services should be personalised and encompass multiple domains, particularly socialising and mobility, and can potentially be delivered by trained non-specialists (Walters *et al.*, 2017). Person-centred care includes all elements, wishes and needs of a person's life that are important to them, not just their symptoms or limitations, which we should accept will change over time.

Governments have recently displayed an increasing interest in utilising behavioural scientific evidence when designing public policy (European Commission, 2016). Health policy is defined by the World Health Organization as 'decisions, plans, and actions that are undertaken to achieve specific health care goals within a society'.[2] Policies are a means for generating and/or supporting the implementation of health behaviour change interventions, which are a set of activities designed to bring about change; thus, policies are crucial for the interventions' implementation and outcomes (Seppälä *et al.*, 2017). Given the sheer diversity of singular and multifaceted frailty interventions, not all of them have been compared in head-to-head studies. Network meta-analyses provide an approach to simultaneous consideration of the relative effectiveness of multiple treatment alternatives (Negm *et al.*, 2017).

A primary concern of aged care policy makers and researchers is to target frailty, and thereby decrease disability, improve functional status and ultimately delay entry into residential aged care facilities (Aggar *et al.*, 2012). As a result, interventions targeting frailty in community-living older people are increasingly being implemented. Health and social care professionals and practitioners have a major task in detecting frail older persons at an early stage in order to avoid unnecessary loss of quality of life and to make timely preventive or curative interventions possible (Gobbens and van Assen, 2014). Developing and implementing interventions must be an essential next step in increasing quality of life of frail older persons. It is important to use peoples' feedback and person-centred outcomes to co-produce improvements in services with those who use them, including the use of targeted interventions. The interventions generally involve referrals, medication and/or dietary changes or monitoring, home visits and exercise programmes, and are strongly influenced by the support of a carer, usually a family member (Pearson *et al.*, 2006; Bouman *et al.*, 2008). In Denmark, national guidelines and payment incentives encourage GPs to provide personal home visits to patients with an age above 75 years and who are considered to be frail (Danish College of General Practitioners, 2012).

Increasing numbers of older citizens worldwide are adding to needs to be addressed by their families, communities and countries, including increased expectations for healthcare, in-home caregiving, and appropriate housing (Crews and Zavotka, 2006). Housing support officers support people who need care and support to help them live independently, find housing and maintain their tenancy. Housing support officers can work in sheltered accommodation, supporting living services, or in the community.[3] As noted elsewhere, however, most older adults are neither frail nor incapable of independent living (e.g. Harper and Crews, 2000). Until recently, studies mainly focused on frailty as a 'non–dynamic entity'. However, frailty can be best understood as a continuum with intermediate states that can be modified, which makes it attractive for preventive public health strategies (Etman *et al.*, 2012). Within the field of health promotion, health is viewed as a resource to handle changes in everyday life (Hartig and Lawrence, 2003). However, a review of health-promotion initiatives targeting older persons highlight the lack of evidence for superiority of one format of intervention over another. The reported value of one particular format, preventive home visits targeting older people in ordinary housing, has varied among different studies (Dahlin-Ivanoff *et al.*, 2016).

Several studies have shown that poor housing conditions in older adults, including lack of basic facilities (i.e. bath or shower), accessibility problems or inadequate indoor temperature control, are associated with worse health outcomes, and higher risk of disease-specific and all-cause mortality. In a recent study, participants with ≥1 poor conditions had a 0.8 per cent higher absolute risk of frailty, a 0.9 per cent higher absolute risk of transportation disability and a 1.34 per cent higher absolute risk of low physical activity per year of follow-up. Given the high prevalence of poor housing, with 52 per cent of the study cohort presenting ≥1 poor condition, these findings have substantial public health relevance (Pérez-Hernández *et al.*, 2018). Prevention programmes targeting functional limitations in older adults should ensure that they live in suitable housing conditions, reflecting a 'joined-up approach'. This requires effective relationships between health and housing providers.

Social health

I have tried very hard in this book to emphasise the critical importance of social health for that person living with frailty. Many social factors have been individually associated with health, including socioeconomic status (measured on both individual and group levels), mastery and control over life circumstances, social support from family and friends, social engagement in group activities, social capital and social cohesion (Andrew and Rockwood, 2010). Conceptualisations of frailty have been categorised as either a 'narrow' approach, focusing on purely medical/physical frailty, or a 'broader' approach that takes into account psychological and social frailty (Van Campen, 2011, p. 15). Whilst these approaches are not mutually exclusive, the conceptualisation and operational definition of frailty within a 'narrow' physical/medical domain has received proportionally more attention in the literature (Nicholson *et al.*, 2013). Social frailty, assessed using simple questions regarding living alone, going out less frequently compared with the prior year, visiting friends sometimes, feeling helpful to friends or family, and talking with someone every day, has a strong impact on the risk of future disability among community-dwelling older people (Makizako *et al.*, 2015). Although frailty is due to an accumulation of deficits in multiple areas such as disease, physical and cognitive impairment, and psychosocial risk factors, previous reviews note that the social and psychological domains of frailty have been neglected (Hogan *et al.*, 2003; Levers *et al.*, 2006).

It is likely that social health will, rightly, become a focus of intervention as well as physical health. 'Social vulnerability' can be broadly understood as the degree to which a person's overall social situation leaves them susceptible to health problems, where 'health problems' are broadly construed to include physical, mental, psychological and functional problems (Andrew and Keefe, 2014).

Overview of interventions

In summary, intervention methods for frail older adults are typically described as including physical exercise, nutritional management, hormone replacement, protein and vitamin D supplementation and lifestyle interventions. Each type of intervention has been shown to have beneficial effects on specific functional parameters in frail older adults (Takano *et al.*, 2016). Likewise, smoking, obesity and inactivity are thought to increase the risk of frailty. Smoking is an important modifiable lifestyle factor and has been examined in population-based studies on frailty. However, in many studies, smoking has been used for adjustment as a confounding covariate to examine independent risks of target outcomes, and only a limited number of studies have focused on associations between smoking and frailty; a recent systematic review provides the evidence of smoking as a predictor of worsening frailty status in a community-dwelling population. Smoking cessation may potentially be beneficial for preventing or reversing frailty (Kojima, Iliffe and Walters, 2015).

Older persons, who are frail and have cognitive impairment, are a clinically important and significant population with a high risk for future adverse health events (Avila-Funes *et al.*, 2009). Once frailty is recognised, opportunities abound for appropriately targeted interventions such as CGAs (Stuck *et al.*, 1993), home-care programmes, or programmes that augment decision making (Moorhouse and Mallery, 2012). Ways to 'manage assets' might include, for example, undertaking a review of polypharmacy for people living with frailty using appropriate tools and in line with current relevant guidance, or to use 'socially prescribed' exercise. Any contemplated intervention will, however, need to be evidence-based, sustainable and tailored to the time constraints and environment of primary and other ambulatory care providers (Muscedere *et al.*, 2016). In older inpatients, frailty might be linked to lower and slower functional recovery. Prospective work is required to confirm these trajectories and understand how to influence them (Hartley *et al.*, 2016).

Mudge and Hubbard (2017) have argued that there are major gaps in our current understanding.

> Large pragmatic implementation trials, co-designed by consumers and inclusive of caregivers, of practical and acceptable community interventions to reduce frailty and its impact. These should be applicable at scale, include longer term clinically meaningful outcomes and thorough cost–benefit analyses.

Interventions could prevent or delay negative health outcomes of frailty for community-dwelling older adults with impacts on family members/caregivers, healthcare providers and the healthcare system. Further, early management of frailty may contribute to improved quality of life for the older adult and their family members/caregivers. As frailty often cannot be averted in persons growing old, its management may lead to better outcomes and delay institutionalisation (Puts *et al.*, 2016).

The recognition of frailty as a long-term condition is a genuinely important issue – a wide range of benefits can be anticipated. Primary care-based registers for frailty could be established and chronic disease models applied systematically for coordinated and person-centred preventative and proactive care. Identifying frailty as a long-term condition would be an important step in distinguishing people with frailty as a discrete population for new research (Harrison *et al.*, 2015).

Introduction to nutritional interventions

There is a link between nutrition and activity, and resilience.

The current literature shows that a number of studies have been conducted to define the relationship between frailty and nutrition. The majority is from cross-sectional, longitudinal and cohort studies. Few intervention studies using micronutrients, macronutrients, nutritional supplement or food regimens have been found. With respect to the nutritional management of pre-frail and frail older people, very few studies have been conducted to determine the effects of protein supplements, either on their own or in combination with exercise. Numerous studies have demonstrated substantial benefits of protein supplementation in combination with resistance exercise in healthy older adults (Jadczak *et al.*, 2017). Finally, various aspects of poor nutritional intake are also considered important biological mechanisms in the development of frailty (Fried *et al.*, 2009; Walston *et al.*, 2006). One sign of impaired nutrition is daily energy intake. The Laboratory of Clinical Epidemiology of the Italian National Research Council of Aging (Florence, Italy) linked calorie intakes of 21 kcal/kg/day or less to frailty (as defined by Fried *et al.*, 2001) in a prospective population-based analysis of 1,155 participants aged 65–102 years (Bartali *et al.*, 2006).

Randomised controlled trials (RCTs) of nutritional interventions in frail individuals remain scarce, although the role of under-nutrition in the frailty process is well-established. Thus, the preventive impact of protein-energy supplementation in frail older adults remains to be proven. One recent RCT included 87 frail community-based adults (usual gait speed <0.6 m/s; Mini Nutritional Assessment <24; mean age, 78 years) with low socioeconomic status (Kim and Lee, 2013). The intervention group received two 200-mL cans of a liquid formula providing 400 kcal, 25 g protein, 9.4 g essential amino acids and 400 mL water per day for 12 weeks, and its impact was compared with a control group who received no supplementation. Overall physical functioning did not change in the control group but improved by 5.9 per cent in the intervention group.

A second RCT assessed the impact of 24 weeks of dietary protein supplementation on muscle mass, strength and physical performance in 65 frail older people, defined by Fried's criteria (Tieland *et al.*, 2012). Muscle strength (leg extension strength) increased from 57.5 to 68.5 kg in the protein group compared with an increase from 57.5 to 63.5 kg in the placebo group. Physical performance (measured with the short physical performance battery) improved significantly from 8.9 to 10.0 of 12 points in the protein group, but did not change in the placebo group (from 7.8 to 7.9 points). Overall, these RCTs favour protein supplementation, which seems to delay or improve the frailty process, as measured by physical performance.

'**Caloric restriction**', arguably, remains the most robust dietary intervention for the extension of lifespan and delay of age-related diseases in diverse species (Barzilai *et al.*, 2012). Few studies have suggested that poor nutrition is related to frailty and that healthy dietary patterns could play a major role in frailty prevention (Kelaiditi *et al.*, 2015).

Dietary interventions

A recent systematic review and meta-analysis shows the first pooled evidence that greater adherence to a Mediterranean diet is associated with significantly lower risk of incident frailty in community-dwelling older people (Kojima *et al.*, 2018). Related topics warranting future research include a focus on which components or combination of foods contributes to the decrease in frailty. Further research is needed to determine whether increasing adherence to a Mediterranean diet can reduce the risk of frailty, including in non-Mediterranean populations (Kojima *et al.*, 2018). There are several potential mechanisms underlying the association between greater adherence to a Mediterranean diet and lower risk of frailty. One possibility is the high intake of foods rich in antioxidants.

An important review by Manal et al. (2015) examined the nutrition intervention studies targeted towards older adults with frailty, and evaluated the effectiveness of nutrition interventions on frailty indicators. The studies were inconsistent in intervention type, duration and targeted outcomes. Most of the studies indicated that modification of nutrition quality, either by giving supplements or by improving diet intake, could improve strength, walking speed, and nutritional status in majority of frail or pre-frail older adults.

Hormonal therapy

Ultimately, the evidence of frailty as a complex system suggests why interventions targeting only one of many dysregulated systems, such as hormonal supplementation, have not been found to prevent or ameliorate frail states (Fried, 2016). For example, many trials of monotherapies, such as replacement of oestrogen or testosterone (e.g. Taaffe et al., 2005; Kenny et al., 2010), for mitigation of frailty have not been successful. There are many other dimensions that need to be understood beyond this; for example, why is it that oestrogen-replacement therapy does not protect against skeletal muscle loss with ageing in women, whereas testosterone does predict muscle mass (Kenny et al., 2003)? Testosterone supplementation may improve muscle mass, muscle strength and physical function in older adults with androgen insufficiency (Sih et al., 1997; Srinivas-Shankar et al., 2010). However, a recent randomised controlled trial was terminated early because of increased cardiovascular adverse events associated with administration of testosterone gel (Basaria et al., 2010). Other potentially effective anabolic hormones included megestrol and growth hormone secretagogues. However, without concurrent exercise training, they tended to increase only muscle mass but not strength or function (Walston et al., 2006).

Exercise and physical activity

The term '**exercise**' defines a planned, structured, repetitive and purposive programme. Exercise training for health and function in older persons contains different components, i.e. strength or power training, aerobic exercise and balance/gait and flexibility training (Montero-Fernandez and Serra-Rexach, 2013; Goisser et al., 2015).

Interventions designed to increase or maintain functional performance, promote physical activity, reduce falls, or enhance wellbeing through reduced anxiety or depression and increased participation may reduce fear of falling. Exercise seems to be a promising intervention to reduce fear of falling since it may directly prevent the decline in physical functioning and mobility (Karinkanta et al., 2012). Besides demonstrated effects on physical performance, there is also evidence regarding beneficial exercise effects on sleep and overall wellbeing (King et al., 1998) Physical exercise is also effective in reducing falls for many individuals with physical risk factors for falls (e.g. impaired strength, balance, functional ability), although the positive effects are less conclusive in frail elderly (Gillespie *et al.*, 2003; Sherrington *et al.*, 2004).

Many reviews and position statements support the benefits of **physical activity** (PA) for function, chronic disease outcomes and mortality benefits in older adults, and these functional benefits extend to frail elders (Bauman *et al.*, 2016). Indeed, only around half of all adults and just a quarter of people aged over 65 years meet the minimum recommended activity levels needed to maintain health (Department of Health, 2011). One has to keep in mind that the term physical activity is used as an umbrella term with different sub-categories, i.e. exercise or leisure time activities (Caspersen *et al.*, 1985). Several systematic reviews regarding physical activity, sometimes even with meta-analyses, have been performed. There is evolving evidence that exercise interventions are important in managing frailty (Freiberger *et al.*, 2016).

The outdoor environment poses a dilemma for older people. On one hand, it offers great opportunities for people to be active, relax and meet people. On the other hand, many activities associated with moving around and enjoying the outdoors require a certain level of strength, agility and stamina, the qualities that many older people are in the process of losing as ageing advances. The term exercise defines a planned, structured, repetitive and purposive programme. Exercise training for health and function in older persons contains different components, i.e. strength or power training, aerobic exercise and balance/gait and flexibility training (Montero-Fernandez and Serra-Rexach, 2013). Important elements of an exercise programme for older persons are volume (e.g. repetition rate in strength training), intensity (how much percentage of the individual capacity) and frequency (e.g. how many exercise sessions per week). Exercise in older persons has beneficial effects and this has led to recommendations for exercise interventions in general for older persons (Chodzko-Zajko *et al.*, 2009). At present, some recommendations are available for frail older persons but they address different components and precise recommendations, e.g. intensity and frequency are lacking.

With an increase in the proportion of older adults, the preventive management of disability in people with multiple chronic conditions and frailty is an important challenge for the health system (Barnett *et al.*, 2012). Disability remains the strongest indicator of frailty even if it does not consistently overlap with frailty (Fried *et al.*, 2001; Gobbens *et al.*, 2010). Frailty is also strongly related to social and economic factors: sometimes disability, particularly moderate disability, can be addressed through social and economic strategies that allow an individual to carry on an independent life despite their physical limitation. Social and economic aspects, such as the presence of a spouse at home or high educational attainment, also act as strong protective factors against frailty, emphasising the need for multidimensional assessment (Liotta *et al.*, 2017). Identifying people with frailty is important in planning healthcare or support interventions; understanding this provides useful information for planning care at the community level since acute healthcare services, including emergency departments, are often considered inappropriate for management of frail patients (Rozzini *et al.*, 2003; Latham and Ackroyd-Stolarz, 2014; Rashwan *et al.*, 2015).

Exercise programmes have been demonstrated to prevent functional and cognitive decline during ageing. In the last decade, the study of exercise programmes exploring their benefits has been mainly focused on community-dwelling older adults, when frailty is identified at an early stage (Rodriguez-Larrad *et al.*, 2017). When compared with control interventions, physical exercise programmes have been shown to reverse frailty and improve cognition, emotional, and social networking in controlled populations of community-dwelling frail older adults (Tarazona-Santabalbina *et al.*, 2016; Pahor *et al.*, 2014). Social networks and communities are beneficial for people living with frailty and their care partners. The concept of frailty is important in helping occupational therapists understand why some elders are more likely to suffer a significant loss of autonomy or need longer hospitalisation after a minor event. Better knowledge about frailty could also mean that occupational therapists can tailor their interventions to the specific and complex needs of this population.

Barriers and goals for PA vary markedly across the life span; they are particularly relevant in the most inactive segment of the population, the oldest-old and frail elderly adults, for whom low PA levels form part of the definition (Baert *et al.*, 2011; Fried *et al.*, 2001). Although attitude toward PA and access to safe and appropriate venues or providers are always important, in the oldest-old and frail adults, individual ability to exercise must also be addressed, as the physical capacity to safely engage in activity is critical to participation, even when attitude and access are not limiting factors. The evidence overall shows that regular physical activity is safe for healthy and for frail older people and the risks of developing major cardiovascular and metabolic diseases, obesity, falls, cognitive impairments, osteoporosis and muscular weakness are decreased by regularly completing activities ranging from low intensity walking through to more vigorous sports and resistance exercises (McPhee *et al.*, 2016). Yet, participation in physical activities remains low amongst older adults, particularly those living in less affluent areas. In addition to falls, ADL disability is of major concern in frail individuals as it is associated with higher rates of mortality (Fried *et al.*, 1998). In the systematic review of 41 studies conducted by Latham, resistance exercise training did not decrease the risk of ADL disability in an elderly population (Latham *et al.*, 2004). In contrast, a Cochrane review of 121 trials found an association between resistance training and reduced ADL disability (Liu and Latham, 2009). Neither review stratified their results by frailty severity.

Multicomponent interventions

Frailty is undeniably a complex health state with multiple domains and dimensions, urging perhaps an approach of **multicomponent interventions**. Other solutions to prevent functional decline are complex interventions, such as preventive home visiting programmes with comprehensive geriatric assessments (Bouman *et al.*, 2008; Gill *et al.*, 2002; Stuck *et al.*, 2002). Little is known about the effectiveness of the different *interacting* components of these complex interventions.

Therefore, to prevent the adverse outcomes of frailty, multicomponent programmes have been implemented and provided a beneficial effect on ADLs and instrumental ADL disability for community-dwelling moderately frail older adults (Daniels *et al.*, 2010). Evaluating the effectiveness of complex interventions within randomised controlled trials is challenging (Blackwood, 2006; Craig *et al.*, 2008; Hawe *et al.*, 2004). Frequently, the intervention is considered effective if a positive result was obtained on the primary outcome. However, to assess the reliability and validity of the trial results, it is important to know the extent to which the intervention was delivered as intended, which is defined as treatment fidelity (Bleijenberg *et al.*, 2016).

Prediction and prevention of disability

There is no consensus on which set of variables should be reliably used to identify older persons at risk of disability in activities of daily living. Physical and psychosocial deficits cluster predominantly into different groups. Even when both are considered simultaneously, the ability to predict incident disability is still insufficient (Costanzo *et al.*, 2017). Published data seem to suggest the fact that a disability state may be independent from morbidity and that women are more disable than men of the same age (Polidoro *et al.*, 2011). The results of a recent prospective cohort study show that physical frailty, even being pre-frail, has a strong impact on increased risk of subsequent disability (Makizako *et al.*, 2015). Among the components of physical frailty, slowness, weakness and weight loss are more strongly associated with incident disability in community-dwelling Japanese older adults. These findings indicate that physical frailty assessments including simple performance measurement (slowness, weakness) and questionnaires (on exhaustion, low activity and weight loss) could be combined for a more effective prediction of disability incidence in the Japanese older population. Frail older adults are often described interchangeably as disabled with multiple chronic diseases (Markle-Reid and Browne, 2003; Topinkova, 2008) because of these concepts' conceptual similarity, co-occurrence and relationship with adverse outcomes (Al Snih *et al.*, 2009).

Disability prevention for older persons, in contrast to disease prevention, has recently been addressed by the Dutch Health Council as function-oriented prevention. The Dutch Health Council emphasises the necessity for development and evaluation of tailor-made interventions that focus on promoting independent functioning in daily life for (vulnerable) older persons with an important role for primary care, screening of vulnerable groups and multidisciplinary cooperation (Daniels *et al.*, 2011). Possibly disability in daily living is a key point of the frailty syndrome and may be the first step for frailty in promoting a substrate for disease and its chronic course (Ahmed *et al.*, 2007).

Care at home

Informal care has been the mainstay of community care for frail older people for many years (Parker, 1990). Overall, there is some evidence that interventions aiming to improve ability to perform independently activities of daily living are effective for a population of homecare service users, in comparison to standard homecare services in which assistance is provided with personal care tasks. However, although there is evidence that these interventions may improve this outcome, there is widespread variation in the type and content of the intervention and the method of evaluation used (Whitehead *et al.*, 2015).

Although homecare has potential to improve this situation, it often focuses on treating disease and 'taking care' of the patient rather than facilitating return to independence. Models of homecare concentrating on optimising function and independence are variously called the 'Active Service Model' (Australia), 'Reablement' (UK) and 'Restorative Home Support' (New Zealand and U.S.) (Parsons *et al.*, 2012). Novel technologies and innovative service provisions aim to maximise the ability to live independently, prevent hospital admissions and address the demand for more efficient health and social care support (Robinson, 2009). Healthcare systems that succeed in preventing long-term care and hospital admissions of frail older people may substantially save on their public spending, but quality indicators of a sufficient methodological level are needed to monitor, compare and improve care quality (Joling *et al.*, 2018). **Reablement** is a time-limited, person-centred, home-based intervention for older people who are at risk of functional decline, often after an accident or period of illness (Glendinning *et al.*, 2010). It aims to help older people to retain, regain or gain skills so that they can manage everyday living skills as independently as possible (Aspinal *et al.*, 2016). There is limited evidence, although not conclusive, that reablement leads to improved function in daily occupations, physical function and health-related quality of life for home-dwelling older adults and to reduced costs and decreased demand for public healthcare services (Tuntland *et al.*, 2016).

Proactive care for frail older people starts with the identification of this group within the community. Research has shown that frailty is related to negative health outcomes, disability and poor quality of life. Reablement is a timely approach to improve homecare services for older people needing care or experiencing functional decline. The healthcare providers are organised into an integrated, coordinated, multidisciplinary team whose members work together with the person towards shared goals (Tinetti *et al.*, 2012). The intervention is targeted, multicomponent and intensive, and takes place in the person's home and local surroundings. The focus is on enhancing performance of daily activities defined as important by the person. The aim is to increase independence in daily activities, and enable people to age in place, be active and participate socially and in the society (Tuntland *et al.*, 2016). From this viewpoint, adequate '**ageing-in-place**' strategies become significantly important. Appropriate and comfortable housing is one of the key determinants to facilitate this desire. One of the aspects of concern is thermal comfort (TC). Many care home residents are old/frail and vulnerable to indoor chilling. A quality indicator for a good 'home' environment is related to TC, a complex interaction involving physiological, social, cultural and clothing factors.[4]

A goal of future work will be to look at groups of users of homecare services and their specific needs For example, in a recent longitudinal analysis involving 5,074 homecare users with intellectual and developmental disabilities in Ontario, increasing age, Down syndrome and living in a group home were significant predictors of deficit accumulation (Ouellette-Kuntz *et al.*, 2018). Rates of deficit accumulation tended to be higher among prefrail and frail individuals; however, impaired cognition and impairment in activities of daily living were associated with slower deficit accumulation.

Equality, independence and communication

Person-centred care for older people living with frailty needs to be specifically related to communication, privacy, personal identity and feelings of vulnerability. Equal access to frailty assessment is important, for example, for people from diverse communities or with specific needs (such as sensory or cognitive impairment). Equality provides evidence for policy makers and professionals to tailor policies and practices to the needs of the older person (Woolhead *et al.*, 2004). In a study of transcripts from interviews with 11 frail older people and 6 informal carers to explore emotion in relation to frailty and deteriorating health, anger and frustration were frequently experienced with declining functional ability towards end of life; sadness occurred with social isolation, loss of autonomy and independence; anxiety was evident when transition to a care home was discussed; and contentment was described when connecting with others (Findlay *et al.*, 2017).

It is important to be able to make a person the focal point of their own care and support, prioritising their wishes and beliefs to support them to retain independence, choice and dignity. The law enforces certain rights. For example, the Care Act 2014 helps to improve people's independence and wellbeing. It makes clear that local authorities must provide or arrange services that help prevent people developing needs for care and support or delay people deteriorating such that they would need ongoing care and support.[5] Equality is an ethical norm to protect against discrimination. It refers to a fundamental aim of justice, namely to ensure fair and equitable treatment. A **human rights approach** to disability means affirming the full personhood of those with mental disabilities by respecting their inherent dignity, their individual autonomy and independence, and their freedom to make their own choices (Burns, 2009). With declining ability and stamina relations with material things, relatives and paid care workers become of central importance for those who have become frail and need assistance with challenges of everyday life (Bjornsdottir, 2017).

Finally, it's important to get the fundamentals right. For example, it is essential to be cognisant of common barriers to communication for people with frailty and the importance of any required support to enable successful communication (e.g. spectacles, hearing aids), or it could be worthy to understand how different customs and preferences, including religious and cultural customs, may impact on communication.

Working with frail older adults is an increasingly important aspect of primary care based practice, and one that requires a sensitive, skilled workforce with effective communication. The challenges for healthcare professionals in recognising frailty among older people are well known alongside the importance of advance care planning, clinician-patient communication and providing appropriate palliative care. To date, communication about frailty with patients and families has received little attention. A NIHR CLAHRC Yorkshire and Humber study[6] is aiming to look at (1) what matters to frail older people, and their informal carers, in their clinical encounters with primary care based practitioners and (2) understand the priorities and challenges for primary care-based practitioners when consulting with frail older people and their informal carers. It is important for the practitioner to understand the principles, processes and options for **self-directed support**,[7] and to be able to support people living with frailty and their families to access self-directed support if so desired. Self-directed support for managing health can, for example, be accessed through people's social networks and engagement with on/offline community resources. CLAHRC Wessex have developed and implemented a social network tool (GENIE) which is being used in a variety of health, social and community settings.[8]

The future

Two burning ways in which we might 'push the pace' are to join up epidemiological and clinical research to identify better target populations for frailty interventions, and to ensure future frailty research studies are redesigned to facilitate rapid implementation into clinical practice (as suggested by Andrew Clegg[9]).

Notes

1 http://thesp.leeds.ac.uk/2015/02/repelling-neoliberal-world-making-aging-dementia-and-iresponse-ability.

2 www.who.int/topics/health_policy/en.

3 www.skillsforcare.org.uk/Careers-in-care/Job-roles/Roles/Housing-support-officer.aspx.

4 www.hra.nhs.uk/planning-and-improving-research/application-summaries/research-summaries/thermal-imaging-in-old-and-frail-in-the-community.

5 www.gov.uk/government/publications/care-act-2014-part-1-factsheets/care-act-factsheets.

6 John Young, Andrew Clegg and Lesley Brown, http://clahrc-yh.nihr.ac.uk/our-themes/primary-care-based-management-of-frailty-in-older-people/projects/5-communication-project.

7 E.g. www.in-control.org.uk/support/support-for-individuals,-family-members-carers/what-is-self-directed-support.aspx.

8 www.clahrc-wessex.nihr.ac.uk/engagement-with-self-directed-support.

9 www.bgs.org.uk/powerpoint/2017spr/clegg_frailty.pdf.

References

Aggar C, Ronaldson S, Cameron ID. (2012). Reactions to caregiving during an intervention targeting frailty in community living older people. *BMC Geriatr.* October 25; 12: 66. doi:10.1186/1471-2318-12-66.

Ahmed N, Mandel R, Fain MJ. (2007). Frailty: an emerging geriatric syndrome. *Am J Med.* 120: 748–53.

Al Snih S, Graham JE, Ray LA, Samper-Ternent R, Markides KS, Ottenbacher KJ. (2009). Frailty and incidence of activities of daily living disability among older Mexican Americans. *J Rehabil Med.* 41: 892–7.

Andrew MK, Keefe JM. (2014). Social vulnerability from a social ecology perspective: a cohort study of older adults from the National Population Health Survey of Canada. *BMC Geriatr.* August 16; 14: 90. doi:10.1186/1471-2318-14-90.

Andrew MK, Rockwood K. (2010). Social vulnerability predicts cognitive decline in a prospective cohort of older Canadians. *Alzheimers Dement.* Jul; 6(4): 319–25.e1. doi:10.1016/j.jalz.2009.11.001.

Apóstolo J, Cooke R, Bobrowicz-Campos E, Santana S, Marcucci M, Cano A, Vollenbroek-Hutten M, Germini F, D'Avanzo B, Gwyther H, Holland C. (2018). Effectiveness of interventions to prevent pre-frailty and frailty progression in older adults: a systematic review. *JBI Database System Rev Implement Rep.* January; 16(1): 140–232. doi:10.11124/JBISRIR-2017-003382.

Aspinal F, Glasby J, Rostgaard T, Tuntland H, Westendorp RG. (2016). New horizons: reablement – supporting older people towards independence. *Age Ageing.* September; 45(5): 572–6. doi:10.1093/ageing/afw094. Epub 2016 May 21.

Avila-Funes JA, Amieva H, Barberger-Gateau P, Le Goff M, Raoux N, Ritchie K, Carrière I, Tavernier B, Tzourio C, Gutiérrez-Robledo LM, Dartigues JF. (2009). Cognitive impairment improves the predictive validity of the phenotype of frailty for adverse health outcomes: the three-city study. *J Am Geriatr Soc.* March; 57(3): 453–61. doi:10.1111/j.1532-5415.2008.02136.x. Epub 2009 February 22.

Baert V, Gorus E, Mets T, Geerts C, Bautmans I. (2011). Motivators and barriers for physical activity in the oldest old: a systematic review. *Ageing Research Reviews.* 10: 464–74. doi:10.1016/j.arr.2011.04.001.

Barnett K, Mercer SW, Norbury M, Watt G, Wyke S, Guthrie B. (2012). Epidemiology of multimorbidity and implications for health care, research, and medical education: across-sectional study, *Lancet.* 380: 37–43.

Bartali B, Frongillo EA, Bandinelli S, Lauretani F, Semba RD, Fried LP, Ferrucci L. (2006). Low nutrient intake is an essential component of frailty in older persons. *Journals of Gerontology. Series A, Biological Sciences and Medical Sciences.* 61: 589–93.

Barzilai N, Huffman DM, Muzumdar RH, Bartke A. (2012). The critical role of metabolic pathways in aging. *Diabetes.* June; 61(6): 1315–22. doi:10.2337/db11-1300.

Basaria S, Coviello AD, Travison TG, Storer TW, Farwell WR, Jette AM et al. (2010). Adverse events associated with testosterone administration. *N Engl J Med.* 363: 109–22.

Bauman A, Merom D, Bull FC, Buchner DM, Fiatarone Singh MA. (2016). Updating the evidence for physical activity: summative reviews of the epidemiological evidence, prevalence, and interventions to promote 'active aging'. *Gerontologist.* April; 56(Suppl. 2): S268–80. doi:10.1093/geront/gnw031.

Bjornsdottir K. (2017). 'Holding on to life': an ethnographic study of living well at home in old age. *Nurs Inq.* December 13. doi:10.1111/nin.12228. [Epub ahead of print].

Blackwood B. (2006). Methodological issues in evaluating complex healthcare interventions. *Journal of Advanced Nursing.* 54(5): 612–22.

Bleijenberg N, Ten Dam VH, Drubbel I, Numans ME, de Wit NJ, Schuurmans MJ. (2016). treatment fidelity of an evidence-based nurse-led intervention in a proactive primary care program for older people. *Worldviews Evid Based Nurs*. February; 13(1): 75–84. doi:10.1111/wvn.12151.

Bouman A, van Rossum E, Evers S, Ambergen T, Kempen G, Knipschild P. (2008). Effects on health care use and associated cost of a home visiting program for older people with poor health status: a randomized clinical trial in the Netherlands. *Journals of Gerontology, Series A, Biological Sciences and Medical Sciences*. 63(3): 291–7.

Burns JK. (2009). Mental health and inequity: a human rights approach to inequality, discrimination, and mental disability. *Health Hum Rights*. 11(2): 19–31.

Caspersen CJ, Powell K, Christenson GM. (1985). Physical activity, exercise, and physical fitness: definitions and distinctions of health-related research. Public Health Rep. 100(2): 126–31.

Chodzko-Zajko WJ, Proctor DN, Fiatarone Singh MA, Minson CT, Nigg CR, Salem GJ et al. (2009). American College of Sports Medicine position stand: exercise and physical activity for older adults. *MedSci Sports Exerc*. 41(7): 1510–30.

Costanzo L, Pedone C, Cesari M, Ferrucci L, Bandinelli S, Antonelli Incalzi R. (2017). Clusters of functional domains to identify older persons at risk of disability. *Geriatr Gerontol Int*. December 28. doi:10.1111/ggi.13226. [Epub ahead of print].

Craig P, Dieppe P, Macintyre S, Michie S, Nazareth I, Petticrew M. (2008). Developing and evaluating complex interventions: the new medical research council guidance. *BMJ*. 337(7676): 979–83.

Crews DE, Zavotka S. (2006). Aging, disability, and frailty: implications for universal design. *Physiol Anthropol*. January; 25(1): 113–8.

Dahlin-Ivanoff S, Eklund K, Wilhelmson K, Behm L, Häggblom-Kronlöf G, Zidén L, Landahl S, Gustafsson S. (2016). For whom is a health-promoting intervention effective? Predictive factors for performing activities of daily living independently. *BMC Geriatr*. October 6; 16(1): 171.

Daniels R, Metzelthin S, van Rossum E, de Witte L, van den Heuvel W. (2010). Interventions to prevent disability in frail community-dwelling older persons: an overview. *Eur J Ageing*. February 9; 7(1): 37–55. doi:10.1007/s10433-010-0141-9. eCollection 2010 March.

Daniels R, van Rossum E, Metzelthin S, Sipers W, Habets H, Hobma S, van den Heuvel W, de Witte L. (2011). A disability prevention programme for community-dwelling frail older persons. *Clin Rehabil*. November; 25(11): 963–74. doi:10.1177/0269215511410728. Epub 2011 August 17.

Danish College of General Practitioners (DSAM). (2012). *Clinical guideline: the elder patient*. Copenhagen.

Department of Health UK (2011). *Start active, stay active: UK. Physical activity guidelines*. Department of Health, UK. www.dh.gov.uk/health/category/publications.

Etman A, Burdorf A, Van der Cammen TJ, Mackenbach JP, Van Lenthe FJ. (2012). Sociodemographic determinants of worsening in frailty among community-dwelling older people in 11 European countries. *J Epidemiol Community Health*. December; 66(12): 1116–21. doi:10.1136/jech-2011-200027. Epub 2012 April 27.

European Commission. (2016). Behavioural insight applied to policy. https://ec.europa.eu/jrc/en/publication/eur-scientific-and-technical-research-reports/behavioural-insights-applied-policy-european-report-2016.

Findlay C, Lloyd A, Finucane AM. (2017). Experience of emotion in frail older people towards the end of life: a secondary data analysis. *Br J Community Nurs*. December 2; 22(12): 586–92. doi:10.12968/bjcn.2017.22.12.586.

Freiberger E, Kemmler W, Siegrist M, Sieber C. (2016). Frailty and exercise interventions: evidence and barriers for exercise programs. *Z Gerontol Geriatr*. October; 49(7): 606–11. Epub 2016 September 21.

Fried LP. (2016). Interventions for human frailty: physical activity as a model. *Cold Spring Harb Perspect Med*. June 1; 6(6). pii: a025916. doi:10.1101/cshperspect.a025916.

Fried LP, Kronmal RA, Newman AB, Bild DE, Mittelmark MB, Polak JF *et al*. (1998). Risk factors for 5-year mortality in older adults: the Cardiovascular Health Study. JAMA. February 25; 279(8): 585–92. [PubMed: 9486752].

Fried LP, Tangen CM, Walston J, Newman AB, Hirsch C, Gottdiener J *et al*. (2001). Frailty in older adults: evidence for a phenotype. *Journals of Gerontology, Series A, Biol Sci Med Sci*. 56A: M146–56.

Fried LP, Xue QL, Cappola AR, Ferrucci L, Chaves P, Varadhan R, Bandeen-Roche K. (2009). Nonlinear multisystem physiological dysregulation associated with frailty in older women: implications for etiology and treatment. *Journals of Gerontology, Series A, Biol Sci Med Sci*. 64: 1049–57.

Frost R, Kharicha K, Jovicic A, Liljas AEM, Iliffe S, Manthorpe J, Gardner B, Avgerinou C, Goodman C, Drennan VM, Walters K. (2017). Identifying acceptable components for home-based health promotion services for older people with mild frailty: a qualitative study. *Health Soc Care Community*. December 5. doi:10.1111/hsc.12526. [Epub ahead of print].

Gill TM, Baker DI, Gottschalk M, Peduzzi PN, Allore H, Byers A. (2002). A program to prevent functional decline in physically frail, elderly persons who live at home. *N Engl J Med*. 347(14): 1068–74.

Gillespie LD, Gillespie WJ, Robertson MC, Lamb SE, Cumming RG, Rowe BH. (2003). Interventions for preventing falls in elderly people. *Cochrane Database Syst Rev*. 4: CD000340.

Glendinning C, Jones K, Baxter K, Rabiee P, Curtis LA, Wilde A, Arksey H, Forder JE. (2010). *Home Care Re-ablement Services: Investigating the longer-term impacts (prospective longitudinal study)*. York: Social Policy Research Unit.

Gobbens RJ, van Assen MA. (2014). The prediction of quality of life by physical, psychological and social components of frailty in community-dwelling older people. *Qual Life Res*. October; 23(8): 2289–300. doi:10.1007/s11136-014-0672-1. Epub 2014 March 27.

Gobbens RJ, Luijkx KG, Wijnen-Sponselee MT, Schols JM. (2010). In search of an integral conceptual definition of frailty: opinions of experts. *Journal of the American Medical Directors Association*. 11(5): 338–43.

Goisser S, Kemmler W, Porzel S, Volkert D, Sieber CC, Bollheimer LC *et al*. (2015). Sarcopenic obesity and complex interventions with nutrition and exercise in community-dwelling older persons: a narrative review. *Clin Interv Aging*. 10: 1267–82.

Gray M, Butler K. (2017). Preventing weakness and stiffness: a top priority for health and social care. *Best Pract Res Clin Rheumatol*. April; 31(2): 255–9. doi:10.1016/j.berh.2017.11.006. Epub 2017 November 17.

Gwyther H, Shaw R, Jaime Dauden EA, D'Avanzo B, Kurpas D, Bujnowska-Fedak M, Kujawa T, Marcucci M, Cano A, Holland C. (2018). Understanding frailty: a qualitative study of European healthcare policy-makers' approaches to frailty screening and management. *BMJ Open*. January 13; 8(1): e018653. doi:10.1136/bmjopen-2017–018653.

Harper GJ, Crews DE. (2000). Aging, senescence, and human variation. In: Stinson S, Huss-Ashmore R, O'Rourke D (eds), *Human biology: an evolutionary and biocultural perspective*. New York: Wiley-Liss, pp. 465–505.

Harrison JK, Clegg A, Conroy SP, Young J. (2015). Managing frailty as a long-term condition. *Age Ageing*. September; 44(5): 732–5. doi:10.1093/ageing/afv085. Epub 2015 July 13.

Hartig T, Lawrence RJ. (2003). Introduction: the residential context of health. *J Soc Issues.* 59(3): 455–73.

Hawe P, Shiell A, Riley T. (2004). Complex interventions: how 'out of control' can a randomised controlled trial be? *BMJ.* 328(7455): 1561.

Hogan DB, MacKnight C, Bergman H. (2003). Models, definitions, and criteria of frailty. *Aging Clin Exp Res.* 15: 1–29.

Jadczak AD, Luscombe-Marsh N, Taylor P, Barnard R, Makwana N, Visvanathan R. (2017). The EXPRESS Study: Exercise and Protein Effectiveness Supplementation Study supporting autonomy in community dwelling frail older people: study protocol for a randomized controlled pilot and feasibility study. *Pilot Feasibility Stud.* July 6; 4: 8. doi:10.1186/s40814-017-0156-5. eCollection 2018.

Joling KJ, van Eenoo L, Vetrano DL, Smaardijk VR, Declercq A, Onder G, van Hout HPJ, van der Roest HG. (2018). Quality indicators for community care for older people: a systematic review. *PLoS One.* January 9; 13(1): e0190298. doi:10.1371/journal.pone.0190298. eCollection 2018.

Karinkanta S, Nupponen R, Heinonen A, Pasanen M, Sievänen H, Uusi-Rasi K, Fogelholm M, Kannus P. (2012). Effects of exercise on health-related quality of life and fear of falling in home-dwelling older women. *J Aging Phys Act.* April; 20(2): 198–214.

Kelaiditi E, Guyonnet S, Cesari M. (2015). Is nutrition important to postpone frailty? *Curr Opin Clin Nutr Metab Care.* January; 18(1): 37–42. doi:10.1097/MCO.0000000000000129.

Kenny AM, Dawson L, Kleppinger A, Iannuzzi-Sucich M, Judge JO. (2003). Prevalence of sarcopenia and predictors of skeletal muscle mass in nonobese women who are long-term users of estrogen-replacement therapy. *J Gerontol A Biol Sci Med Sci.* 58: M436–40.

Kenny AM, Kleppinger A, Annis K, Rathier M, Browner B, Judge JO, McGee D. (2010). Effects of transdermal testosterone on bone and muscle in older men with low bioavailable testosterone levels, low bone mass, and physical frailty. *J Am Geriatr Soc.* 58: 1134–43.

Kim C-O, Lee K-R. (2013). Preventive effect of protein-energy supplementation on the functional decline of frail older adults with low socioeconomic status: a community based randomized controlled study. *J Gerontol A Biol Sci Med Sci.* 68(3): 309–16.

King AC, Rejeski WJ, Buchner DM. (1998). Physical activity interventions targeting older adults: a critical review and recommendations. *Am J Prev Med.* 15: 316–33.

Kojima G, Avgerinou C, Iliffe S, Walters K. (2018). Adherence to Mediterranean diet reduces incident frailty risk: systematic review and meta-analysis. *J Am Geriatr Soc.* January 11. doi:10.1111/jgs.15251. [Epub ahead of print].

Kojima G, Iliffe S, Walters K. (2015). Smoking as a predictor of frailty: a systematic review. *BMC Geriatr.* October 22; 15: 131. doi:10.1186/s12877-015-0134-9. Review.

Latham L, Ackroyd-Stolarz S. (2014). Emergency dept utilization by older adults: a descriptive study. *Can Geriatr J.* December; 17(4): 118–25. http://dx.doi.org/10.5770/cgj.17.108 [Published online 2014 December 2].

Latham NK, Bennett DA, Stretton CM, Anderson CS. (2004). Systematic review of progressive resistance strength training in older adults. *J Gerontol A Biol Sci Med Sci.* January; 59(1): 48–61. [PubMed: 14718486].

Levers MJ, Estabrooks CA, Ross Kerr JC. (2006). Factors contributing to frailty: literature review. *J Adv Nurs.* 56: 282–91.

Liotta G, O'Caoimh R, Gilardi F, Proietti MG, Rocco G, Alvaro R, Scarcella P, Molloy DW, Orlando S, Mancinelli S, Palombi L, Stievano A, Marazzi MC. (2017). Assessment of frailty in community-dwelling older adults residents in the Lazio region (Italy): a model to plan regional community-based services. *Arch Gerontol Geriatr.* January–February; 68: 1–7. doi:10.1016/j.archger.2016.08.004. Epub 2016 August 12.

Liu CJ, Latham NK. (2009). Progressive resistance strength training for improving physical function in older adults. *Cochrane Database Syst Rev.* 3: CD002759. [PubMed: 19588334].

Makizako H, Shimada H, Doi T, Tsutsumimoto K, Suzuki T. (2015). Impact of physical frailty on disability in community-dwelling older adults: a prospective cohort study. *BMJ Open.* September 2; 5(9): e008462. doi:10.1136/bmjopen-2015-008462.

Manal B, Suzana S, Singh DK. (2015). Nutrition and frailty: a review of clinical intervention studies. *J Frailty Aging.* 4(2): 100–6. doi:10.14283/jfa.2015.49.

Manton KG. (1988). A longitudinal study of functional change and mortality in the United States. *J Gerontol.* 43: 153–61.

Markle-Reid M, Browne G. (2003). Conceptualization of frailty in relation to older adults. *J Adv Nurs.* 44: 58–68.

McGuigan FE, Bartosch P, Åkesson KE. (2017). Musculoskeletal health and frailty. *Best Pract Res Clin Rheumatol.* April; 31(2): 145–59. doi:10.1016/j.berh.2017.11.002. Epub 2017 November 20.

McPhee JS, French DP, Jackson D, Nazroo J, Pendleton N, Degens H. (2016). Physical activity in older age: perspectives for healthy ageing and frailty. *Biogerontology.* June; 17(3): 567–80. doi:10.1007/s10522-016-9641-0. Epub 2016 March 2.

Montero-Fernandez N, Serra-Rexach JA. (2013). Role of exercise on sarcopenia in the elderly. *Eur J Phys Rehabil Med.* 49(1): 131–43.

Moorhouse P, Mallery LH. (2012). Palliative and therapeutic harmonization: a model for appropriate decision making in frail older adults. *J Am Ger Soc.* 60(12): 2326–32.

Mudge AM, Hubbard RE. (2017) Frailty: mind the gap. *Age Ageing.* https://doi.org/10.1093/ageing/afx193. [Epub ahead of print].

Muscedere J, Andrew MK, Bagshaw SM, Estabrooks C, Hogan D, Holroyd-Leduc J, Howlett S, Lahey W, Maxwell C, McNally M, Moorhouse P, Rockwood K, Rolfson D, Sinha S, Tholl B; Canadian Frailty Network (CFN). (2016). Screening for frailty in Canada's health care system: a time for action. *Can J Aging.* September; 35(3): 281–97. doi:10.1017/S0714980816000301. Epub 2016 May 23.

Negm AM, Kennedy CC, Thabane L, Veroniki AA, Adachi JD, Richardson J, Cameron ID, Giangregorio A, Papaioannou A. (2017). Management of frailty: a protocol of a network meta-analysis of randomized controlled trials. *Syst Rev.* July 5; 6(1): 130. doi:10.1186/s13643-017-0522-7.

Nicholson C, Meyer J, Flatley M, Holman C, Van Campen, C. (2011). Frail older persons in the Netherlands. The Netherlands Institute for Social Research, The Hague, Netherlands.

Nicholson C, Meyer J, Flatley M, Holman C. (2013). The experience of living at home with frailty in old age: a psychosocial qualitative study. *Int J Nurs Stud.* September; 50(9): 1172–9. doi:10.1016/j.ijnurstu.2012.01.006. Epub 2012 February 4.

Ouellette-Kuntz H, Martin L, McKenzie K. (2018). Rate of deficit accumulation in home care users with intellectual and developmental disabilities. *Ann Epidemiol.* January 31. pii: S1047–2797(17)30586–0. doi:10.1016/j.annepidem.2018.01.010. [Epub ahead of print].

Pahor M, Guralnik JM, Ambrosius WT, Blair S, Bonds DE, Church TS *et al.* (2014). Effect of structured physical activity on prevention of major mobility disability in older adults: the LIFE study randomized clinical trial. *JAMA.* 311(23): 2387–96. doi:10.1001/jama.2014.5616.

Parker G. (1990). *With due care and attention: a review of research on informal care.* Occasional Paper No 2. London: Family Policy Studies Centre.

Parsons J, Rouse P, Robinson EM, Sheridan N, Connolly MJ. (2012). Goal setting as a feature of homecare services for older people: does it make a difference? *Age Ageing.* January; 41(1): 24–9. doi:10.1093/ageing/afr118. Epub 2011 September 6.

Pearson S, Inglis SC, McLennan, Brennan L, Russell M, Wilkinson D, Thompson DR, Stewart S. (2006). Prolonged effects of a home-based intervention in patients with chronic illness. *Arch Intern Med.* 166(6): 645–50.

Pérez-Hernández B, Lopez-García E, Graciani A, Ayuso-Mateos JL, Rodríguez-Artalejo F, García-Esquinas E. (2018). Housing conditions and risk of physical function limitations: a prospective study of community-dwelling older adults. *J Public Health* (Oxf). January 17. doi:10.1093/pubmed/fdy004. [Epub ahead of print].

Puts MT, Toubasi S, Atkinson E, Ayala AP, Andrew M, Ashe MC, Bergman H, Ploeg J, McGilton KS. (2016). Interventions to prevent or reduce the level of frailty in community-dwelling older adults: a protocol for a scoping review of the literature and international policies. *BMJ Open.* March 2; 6(3): e010959. doi:10.1136/bmjopen-2015-010959.

Rashwan W, Abo-Hamad W, Arisha A. (2015). A system dynamics view of the acute bed blockage problem in the Irish Healthcare System. *European Journal of Operational Research.* 247(1): 276–93.

Robinson P. (2009). *Are hospital admissions out of control?* Alcester, Warwickshire: Caspe Healthcare Knowledge Systems.

Rodríguez-Larrad A, Arrieta H, Rezola C, Kortajarena M, Yanguas JJ, Iturburu M, Susana MG, Irazusta J. (2017). Effectiveness of a multicomponent exercise program in the attenuation of frailty in long-term nursing home residents: study protocol for a randomized clinical controlled trial. *BMC Geriatr.* February 23; 17(1): 60. doi:10.1186/s12877-017-0453-0.

Rozzini R, Sabatini T, Trabucchi M. (2003). The network of elderly care in Italy: only a correct use of acute ward allows an overall functioning of the health care system. *Journal of Gerontology: Medical Sciences.* 58A(2): 190–1.

Seppälä T, Hankonen N, Korkiakangas E, Ruusuvuori J, Laitinen J. (2017). National policies for the promotion of physical activity and healthy nutrition in the workplace context: a behaviour change wheel guided content analysis of policy papers in Finland. *BMC Public Health.* August 2; 18(1): 87. doi:10.1186/s12889-017-4574-3.

Sherrington C, Lord SR, Finch CF. (2004). Physical activity interventions to prevent falls among older people: update of the evidence. *J Sci Med Sport.* 7: 43–51.

Sih R, Morley JE, Kaiser FE, Perry 3rd HM, Patrick P, Ross C. (1997). Testosterone replacement in older hypogonadal men: a 12-month randomized controlled trial. *J Clin Endocrinol Metab.* 82: 1661–7.

Srinivas-Shankar U, Roberts SA, Connolly MJ, O'Connell MD, Adams JE, Oldham JA et al. (2010). Effects of testosterone on muscle strength, physical function, body composition, and quality of life in intermediate-frail and frail elderly men: a randomized, double-blind, placebo-controlled study. *J Clin Endocrinol Metab.* 95: 639–50.

Stuck AE, Egger M, Hammer A, Minder CE, Beck JC. (2002). Home visits to prevent nursing home admission and functional decline in elderly people: systematic review and meta-regression analysis. *JAMA.* 287(8): 1022–8.

Stuck AE, Siu AL, Wieland GD, Adams J, Rubenstein LZ. (1993). Comprehensive geriatric assessment: a meta-analysis of controlled trials. *Lancet.* October 23; 342(8878): 1032–6.

Taaffe DR, Sipila S, Cheng S, Puolakka J, Toivanen J, Suominen H. (2005). The effect of hormone replacement therapy and/or exercise on skeletal muscle attenuation in postmenopausal women: a yearlong intervention. *Clin Physiol Funct Imaging.* 25: 297–304.

Takano E, Teranishi T, Watanabe T, Ohno K, Kitaji S, Sawa S, Kanada Y, Toba K, Kondo I. (2016). Differences in the effect of exercise interventions between prefrail older adults and older adults without frailty: a pilot study. *Geriatr Gerontol Int.* August 21. doi:10.1111/ggi.12853. [Epub ahead of print].

Tarazona-Santabalbina FJ, Gómez-Cabrera MC, Pérez-Ros P, Martínez-Arnau FM, Cabo H, Tsaparas K et al. (2016). A multicomponent exercise intervention that reverses frailty and improves cognition, emotion, and social networking in the community-dwelling frail elderly: a randomized clinical trial. *J Am Med Dir Assoc.* 17(5): 426–33. doi:10.1016/j.jamda.2016.01.019.

Tieland M, van de Rest O, Dirks ML, van der Zwaluw N, Mensink M, van Loon LJ, de Groot LC. (2012). Protein supplementation improves physical performance in frail elderly people: a randomized, double-blind, placebo-controlled trial. *J Am Med Dir Assoc.* October; 13(8): 720–6. doi:10.1016/j.jamda.2012.07.005. Epub 2012 August 11.

Tinetti ME, Charpentier P, Gottschalk M, Baker DI. (2012). Effect of a restorative model of posthospital home care on hospital readmissions. *J Am Geriatr Soc.* 60(8): 1521–6.

Topinkova E. (2008). Aging disability and frailty. *Ann Nutr Metab.* 52(Suppl. 1): 6–11.

Tuntland H, Kjeken I, Langeland E, Folkestad B, Espehaug B, Førland O, Aaslund MK. (2016). Predictors of outcomes following reablement in community-dwelling older adults. *Clin Interv Aging.* December 29; 12: 55–63. doi:10.2147/CIA.S125762. eCollection 2017.

Van Campen C. (2011). *Frail older persons in the Netherlands.* The Hague, Netherlands: Netherlands Institute for Social Research.

Walston J, Hadley EC, Ferrucci L, Guralnik JM, Newman AB, Studenski SA *et al.* (2006). Research agenda for frailty in older adults: toward a better understanding of physiology and etiology. Summary from the American Geriatrics Society/National Institute on Aging Research Conference on Frailty in Older Adults. *J Am Geriatr Soc.* 54: 991–1001.

Walters K, Frost R, Kharicha K, Avgerinou C, Gardner B, Ricciardi F, Hunter R, Liljas A, Manthorpe J, Drennan V, Wood J, Goodman C, Jovicic A, Iliffe S. (2017). Home-based health promotion for older people with mild frailty: the HomeHealth intervention development and feasibility RCT. *Health Technol Assess.* December; 21(73): 1–128. doi:10.3310/hta21730.

Whitehead PJ, Worthington EJ, Parry RH, Walker MF, Drummond AE. (2015). Interventions to reduce dependency in personal activities of daily living in community dwelling adults who use homecare services: a systematic review. *Clin Rehabil.* November; 29(11): 1064–76. doi:10.1177/0269215514564894. Epub 2015 January 13.

Woolhead G, Calnan M, Dieppe P, Tadd W. (2004). Dignity in older age: what do older people in the United Kingdom think? *Age Ageing.* March; 33(2): 165–70.

7

PERSON-CENTRED INTEGRATED CARE AND END OF LIFE

Aim

People living with frailty and their care partners need support to live, but need proper care at the right time, in the right place, in the right way. Practitioners in frailty need to understand what is truly important to people, and to make sure people's needs are met, whether in health, social care, housing or beyond. The complexity of people who are frail itself means that persons cannot only be defined by a diagnostic label, and the future direction of promoting health and wellbeing is undoubtedly challenging.

Introduction

There is huge potential for frailty to be managed in a more integrated and person-centred manner; there is also a need to raise its profile and develop a common understanding of it among stakeholders, as well as consistency in how and when it is measured (Gwyther *et al.*, 2018). **Person-centred care** that focuses on respecting the person's identity, creating relationships and sharing decision making is important to provide high-quality care (NIHR Dissemination Centre, 2017). Healthcare systems internationally are facing the challenges of providing care to an ageing population (Christensen *et al.*, 2009).

Population ageing will be the major driver of projected increases in disease burden in older people, most evident in low-income and middle-income countries and for strongly age-dependent disorders (for example, dementia, stroke, chronic obstructive pulmonary disease and diabetes). These are also the disorders for which chronic disability makes a substantial contribution to burden (Cesari *et al.*, 2016). Even though older adults living with frailty are significant users of healthcare resources, their input remains under-represented in research, healthcare decision making and health policy formulation. As such, engaging older adults living with frailty and their family caregivers is not only an ethical imperative, but their input is imperative as health and social care systems evolve from a single-illness model to one which accounts for the complex and chronic needs that accompany frailty (Holroyd-Leduc *et al.*, 2016).

Frailty is recognised as a 'life-limiting condition', strongly associated with increased patient mortality, comorbidity, longer periods of hospitalisation and repeat admissions (Karunananthan *et al.*, 2009; Clegg *et al.*, 2013). Several factors make development of a policy on ageing so difficult. It is argued that the critical component of the policy on ageing is **a life–course perspective**. This recognises, first, that life experiences powerfully shape how people grow old and, second, that these experiences are socially rather than biologically constructed (Dannefer, 2003; Walker, 2006). Approximately 25 per cent of the heterogeneity in health and function in older age is genetically determined, with the remainder strongly affected by the cumulative effect of health behaviours and inequities across the life course (Beard and Bloom, 2015). Interactions of different aspects of an individual's life are dynamic and vulnerabilities in some areas of a person's life might be overcome by promoting resilience on other areas. In contrast, someone born into a poor family with limited access to education, or in a marginalised cultural group, is likely to have poor health in older age and earlier mortality (e.g. World Health Organization Europe, 2010). A person's 'life story', including their individual cultural and religious background, can offer insight into their priorities and wellbeing. 'Life story work' is an activity in which the person with dementia is supported by staff and family members to gather and review their past life events and build a personal biography. It may help challenge ageist attitudes and assumptions, be used as a basis for personalised care, improve assessment, assist in transitions between different care environments, and help to develop improved relationships between care staff and family carers (McKeown *et al.*, 2006). It is used to help the person make some sense of their past experiences and how they have coped with events in their life. Life story work can help encourage better communication and an understanding of the person's needs and wishes. This can inform their care and ensure that it is provided in a positive and person-centred way.

Service improvement, integrated care pathways and co-production

There is often some confusion as to whether a project falls within the realms of audit, research or evaluation. An evaluation is

> a process that takes place before, during and after an activity. It includes looking at the quality of the content, the delivery process and the impact of the activity or programme on the audience(s) or participants. It is concerned with making an assessment, judging an activity or service against a set of criteria. Evaluation assesses the worth or value of something.[1]

It is worth noting clear differences between clinical audit, research and evaluation:

- **clinical audit** measures existing practice against evidence-based clinical standards. All clinical audit must comply with clinical audit governance requirements.
- **research** generates new knowledge that has the potential to be generalisable or transferable. All research must comply with research governance requirements.
- **evaluation** is designed to support service improvement and it should always be well connected to action. It will *not* produce new generalisable or transferable knowledge.

It is further important to share findings of research, audit or evaluation clearly and accurately in written or verbal form; all practitioners need to participate regularly in continuing professional development to ensure the investigation methods used are robust, valid and reliable. A goal should be to disseminate and promote new and evidence-based practice continually, and challenge poor practice. It is worth reviewing the main community-based interventions we have evaluated and their impact, and identify points that may help those designing, implementing and evaluating such interventions in future. As an overview of the whole system, the research summary, 'Evaluating integrated and community-based care: how do we know what works?', published by the Nuffield Trust in June 2013,[2] was a useful contribution. It is, however, especially worth noting the outcomes and experience measures reported by people living with frailty, their families and care partners.

When a frail older person requires admission to hospital, best practice models such as those employed by Sheffield Teaching Hospitals Trust should be adopted systematically (Health Foundation, 2013). This includes 'discharge to assess', where patients are discharged once they are medically fit and have an assessment with the appropriate members of the social care and community intermediate care teams in their own home (NHS England, 2014). A proposed framework of an 'integrated care pathway', which targets healthy seniors as well as those with disabilities or chronic illnesses, takes account of all the intervention factors and strategies intended to maintain or improve the health of an older person (Dubuc *et al.*, 2013). The proposed model includes nine main focuses of intervention. The first five (1–5 in Figure 7.1) involve action on the main health determinants; the other four (6–9), on risk factors and health conditions through the prevention of specific problems and the optimisation of remaining abilities in the population concerned.

Pathways of care to meet the needs of people living with frailty and those important to them consider the common acute presentations, including frailty syndromes. Excellent care pathways, with a 'joined up' 'whole systems' approach have been developed locally for frailty (see, for example, the Northumberland pathway,[3] which is noteworthy because of its involvement of patients and care partners in the co-design).

NHS England produced an excellent document in February 2014, 'Safe, compassionate care for frail older people using an integrated care pathway: practical guidance for commissioners, providers and nursing, medical and allied health

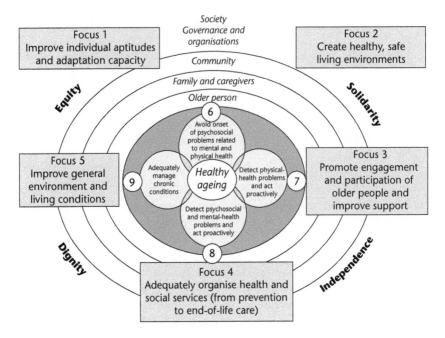

FIGURE 7.1 Healthy ageing conceptual model

Source: reproduced under copyright through Creative Commons License, from Figure 2 of Dubuc N, Bonin L, Tourigny A, Mathieu L, Couturier Y, Tousignant M, Corbin C, Delli-Colli N, Raîche M. (2013). Development of integrated care pathways: toward a care management system to meet the needs of frail and disabled community-dwelling older people. *Int J Integr Care*. May 17; 13: e017. Print 2013 April.

professional leaders'.[4] The frailty pathway and tools set out in this guidance have the potential to reduce harm and improve the experience of older people, and implementation of this pathway underpins all five domains of the NHS Outcomes Framework. It is designed to engage and capture the energies and commitment of medical, nursing and allied health professional leaders who have responsibility for meeting the domain requirements.

The practitioner is expected to value collaborative involvement and co-production with people to improve person-centred design and quality of services. In a blogpost from NHS England dated 26 November 2015, NHS England's National Clinical Director for Long Term Conditions looked at what co-production means to the Long Term Conditions Unit and how it is essential to supporting person-centred care.[5]

Martin McShane comments that 'Co-production is a way of working. It's about equal partnerships – services and organisations working together with patients, carers, families and service users to co-design care and support.' If frail older people are supported in living independently and understanding their long-term conditions, and educated to manage them effectively, they are less likely to reach crisis, require urgent care support and experience harm (NHS England, 2014). There is evidence of seasonal peaks during winter, partly explained by similar patterns in admission spells (Soong *et al.*, 2015).

With an ageing population, significant financial challenges and a potentially fragmented health and social care system, the issue of the appropriateness of emergency admission is a pressing one which requires further research, greater focus on the experiences of older people and their families, and more nuanced contextual and evidence-based responses (Thwaites *et al.*, 2017).

> As people get older, they have more things wrong with them. And the more things they have wrong with them, the more likely they are to die. But everyone accumulates deficits at a different rate, and not all people of the same age have the same short-term risk of dying. This variable susceptibility to death and other adverse outcomes in older people of the same age is called frailty.
>
> *(Koller and Rockwood, 2013, p. 168)*

Disease trajectories

Conceptualising frailty as a continuum implies a dynamic or changing trajectory. The 'frailty trajectory' is characterised by poor long-term functional status and a slow decline with no clear terminal phase. This group is likely to include older people with dementia, frailty and multiple morbidity, and often requires months or years of years of supportive and health services input before death (Walsh *et al.*, 2012). In summary, frailty tends to follow a trajectory of progressive disability from an already low baseline of cognitive or physical functioning (Murray *et al.*, 2005). This trajectory may be cut short by death after an acute event such as a fractured neck or femur, or pneumonia.

Disease trajectories typically vary (see Figure 7.2).

Trajectory A: short period of evident decline, typically cancer
This entails a reasonably predictable decline in physical health over a period of weeks, months or, in some cases, years.

Trajectory B: long term limitations with intermittent serious episodes
With conditions such as heart failure and chronic obstructive pulmonary disease, patients are usually ill for many months or years with occasional acute, often severe, exacerbations. Deteriorations are generally associated.

Trajectory C: 'prolonged dwindling'
People who escape cancer and organ system failure are likely to die at an older age of either brain failure (such as dementia) or frailty.

Disease trajectories typically vary.

Location on the continuum of frailty is critical to determining the degree of vulnerability of the older adult and the type of interventions that are needed (Espinoza

function

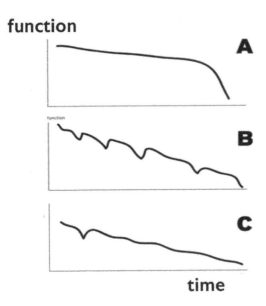

FIGURE 7.2 Disease trajectories

and Walston, 2005). Patients with advanced frailty, with or without cognitive impairment, have an end of life functional course marked by slowly progressive functional deterioration, with only a slight acceleration in the trajectory of functional loss as death approaches. Patients with cognitive impairment have particularly high rates of functional impairment at the time of death (Covinsky *et al.*, 2003). These results suggest that end of life care systems that are targeted toward patients with functional trajectories clearly suggesting impending death are poorly suited to older people dying with progressive frailty. People living with frailty tend to have the lowest rate of functional decline in the last year of life (Cohen-Mansfield *et al.*, 2017).

In a fascinating recent study, all 34 participants, older people living with frailty approaching end of life, completed interviews which reported a gradual physical decline and a diminishing social world from already low levels (Lloyd *et al.*, 2016). Psychological and existential wellbeing dipped in response to changes in circumstances or periods of physical or emotional illness. Wellbeing related to whether the older person was able to adapt to their new situation. Some reached a tipping point where carers were unable to continue to support the older people to live in the way that reflected their sense of self. They then experienced increasing psychological and existential distress with a **social death** prior to dying (see Borgstrom, 2017 for an excellent discussion of 'social death'). Frail older people's sense of meaning and purpose in life remained steady in the coping narrative but eroded gradually and finally in the other scenarios.

Person-centred integrated care and frailty

Effective integrated working across health, social care, community and voluntary sectors is important to optimise patient or population care for people living with frailty. Inter-professional and multi-agency collaboration may include, for example, primary care, ambulance service, fire and rescue service, police, housing, geriatricians, old-age psychiatrists and palliative care clinical nurse specialists. Integrated care is increasingly perceived as an important way to reorganise care for the frail elderly. The person-centredness can be emphasised if integrated care is defined as 'a well planned and well organised set of services and care processes, targeted at multidimensional needs and problems of an individual client, or a category of persons with similar needs/problems' (Looman *et al.*, 2016).

As a result of changing patterns in the demand for healthcare, healthcare systems are being compelled to embrace person-centred and integrated care services. These still evolving services enable healthcare systems to provide a continuum of modern self-management support, and age specific, coherent, proactive and preventive care and support. It may sometimes be necessary to share information, including that which relates to a person's wishes, in a timely and appropriate manner with those involved in a person's care, considering issues of confidentiality and ensuring that where information is already available, the person is not asked to provide the same information repeatedly. Person-centred and integrated care services are based on the needs and expectations of persons and their informal network, and not only on diseases (Uittenbroek *et al.*, 2016). This is especially important to ensure that people living with frailty do not feel anonymised within the system (which is why campaigns such as '#hellomynameis'[2] can be so empowering for patients). For example, it is noted that

> The process of becoming an in-patient can lead to loss of identity for patients, particularly if they have dementia. Findings showed that older patients need to be able to remember and relate to important people, events and things, and staff knowing about their life context, such as family and occupation, can help with this.
>
> *(Bridges* et al., *2010, p. 93)*

Patient–centeredness, therefore, has become a legitimate base for healthcare provision, and has been reinforced by laws that strengthen patient's rights (Fabbricotti *et al.*, 2013). The prevailing belief, for example, in the United States might be that integrated care has the capacity to solve many of problems by improving care coordination and continuity; streamlining disjointed services and systems; eliminating duplication; reducing administrative and service costs; and promoting more equitable distribution of resources (Kodner and Kyriacou, 2000). Based on the literature on integrated care covering the period from 1997 to 2010 inclusive, it appears that there are essentially two types of models of integrated care delivery for the frail elderly:

One type of model is a smaller, community-based model which relies on cooperation across care providers, focused on home and community care, but the second type of model is a larger-scale model which has a single administrative authority and a single budget and which includes both home/community and residential services.

(Béland and Hollander, 2013)

The emphasis on 'care coordination' (or 'care navigation') for the delivery of person-centred care can never be underestimated, despite nuances in the exact definition, for example:

There is no universal definition of care navigation or a 'care navigator'; navigation at its heart is a coordination process and key ingredient to achieve integrated care provision to improve health and well-being. A person providing in care navigation is usually based in a multidisciplinary team, helps identify and signpost people to available services, acting as link workers.

(Health Education England, 'Care navigation: a competency framework', p.6)[6]

In developed countries, health systems are pressured to reconsider the restructuring of services provided to new clusters of patients with complex needs, as growth in clinical specialisation – due to the rapid expansion of medical knowledge and technologies – tends to fragment patient care. Integrated care initiatives endeavour to align healthcare provision with evolving patient needs (Calciolari and Ilinca, 2016). Modern healthcare systems have largely been designed around single-organ disease-based services, with increasing specialism notable within hospital care. Historically, this has also been reflected in primary care, because general practitioner incentivisation schemes, such as the UK Quality and Outcomes Framework, are constructed using disease-based targets, and clinical guidelines are usually designed around single long-term conditions (Turner *et al.*, 2014).

Frail older people themselves prefer to grow old in the community and want to live independently at home as long as possible; also referred to as **'ageing in place'** (Looman *et al.*, 2016). Frail older people often require tailored rehabilitation in order to remain at home, especially following a period of hospitalisation. Restorative care services aim to enhance an older person's ability to remain or improve physical functioning, either at home or in residential care, but evidence of their effectiveness is limited. Senior and colleagues (2014) found that restorative care models that utilise case management and multidisciplinary care may positively impact on institution-free survival for frail older people without adversely impacting on the health of caregivers. The current workforce of physicians, nurses and skilled rehabilitation professionals is allegedly one-tenth of that ideally required (thus 'The need to scale up rehabilitation').[7]

Multidisciplinary team members can predict each patient's rehabilitation potential to maximise best use of resources. A crucial question surrounds rehabilitation following hospital admission. The study, known as HERO (Home-based Extended

Rehabilitation of Older people), will involve 718 older people with frailty admitted to hospital following acute illness or injury. The HERO trial[8] hopefully will provide robust evidence on the clinical and cost-effectiveness of a home-based exercise intervention as extended rehabilitation for older people with frailty following discharge from hospital. The trial has chosen quality of life as our main outcome of importance for older people, and will also collect detailed information on health and social care resource use.

A central message is that traditional 'disease-specific' care delivery models do not fit well with the comprehensive and complex needs of people with multimorbidity and frailty. Efficient and preferably cost-effective approaches of care delivery are therefore urgently needed (Hopman *et al.*, 2016). There are limitations to frailty/risk-stratification tools in the urgent care context: although most scales performed better than chance in predicting a range of poor outcomes, none of them performed adequately for individual clinical decision making (Conroy and Dowsing, 2013). Risk-stratifying older people accessing urgent care is a potentially useful first step to ensuring that the most vulnerable are able to access optimal care from the start of the episode. While there are many risk-stratification tools reported in the literature, few have addressed the practical issues of implementation (Elliott *et al.*, 2017). Generally, redesigning the system of care for older emergency patients led to reductions in bed occupancy and mortality without affecting readmission rates or requiring additional resources (Silvester *et al.*, 2014).

Given the detrimental physical and psychological impact of frailty on older people, as well as its potential mitigation or even reversibility, frailty may be a promising target of interventions. Frail older people, who are not highly fit but not completely disabled, are the population likely to benefit most from such interventions (Kojima *et al.*, 2017). Societies worldwide are challenged by the ongoing growth in healthcare expenditures and the changing patterns in the demand for healthcare. Long-term care expenditures continue to grow and are expected to double within the coming decades and the number of elderly people with multiple chronic conditions is increasing drastically (Spoorenberg *et al.*, 2013). The **WHO Framework on integrated people-centred health services** is a call for a fundamental shift in the way health services are funded, managed and delivered.[9] It supports countries progress towards universal health coverage by shifting away from health systems designed around diseases and health institutions towards health systems designed for people (see Figure 7.3).

There have been a number of significant '**barriers to integrated care**', for example a cultural bias within specialities and primary care to considering 'one disease at a time', viewing non-communicable diseases as lesser importance than transmissible or infectious diseases.[10] Despite indications that comprehensive care programmes for multimorbid patients decrease inpatient healthcare utilisation and healthcare costs, improve health behaviour of patients and perceived quality of care, and realise satisfaction of patients and caregivers because of the heterogeneity of the programmes, it is as yet too early to draw firm conclusions regarding their effectiveness (de Bruin *et al.*, 2012). The performance of healthcare organisations is routinely

Strategy 1: Engaging and empowering people and communities

Engaging and empowering individuals and families
Engaging and empowering communities
Engaging and empowering informal carers
Reaching the underserved and marginalised

Strategy 2: Strengthening governance and accountability

Bolstering participatory governance
Enhancing mutual accountability

Strategy 3: Reorienting the model of care

Defining service priorities based on life-course needs, respecting social preferences
Revaluing promotion, prevention and public health
Building strong primary-care systems
Shifting towards more outpatient and ambulatory care
Innovating and incorporating new technologies

Strategy 4: Coordinating services within and across sectors

Coordinating care for individuals
Coordinating health programmes and providers
Coordinating across sectors

Strategy 5: Creating an enabling environment

Strengthening leadership and management for change
Strengthening information systems and knowledge
Striving for quality improvement and safety
Reorienting the health workforce
Aligning regulatory frameworks
Improving funding and reforming payment systems

FIGURE 7.3 WHO Framework on integrated people-centred health services

Source: adapted from www.who.int/servicedeliverysafety/areas/people-centred-care/Over view_IPCHS_final.pdf.

assessed, whether by payers, governments, or by organisations representing patients. Patient experience is an important outcome of healthcare, and surveys to measure patient experience are now widely used to assess care quality (Lyratzopoulos *et al.*, 2011).

There is a number of factors which are considered very important for making integrated care work, also applicable to frailty. These are shown in Box 7.1.

Although advances in assistive technology (AT) and the delivery of preventative care are relevant to many older adults, when frailty or dementia are present, individualised care planning is especially critical to ensure that 'standard of care' interventions for each health concern align with overall goals of care and prognosis (Moorhouse and Mallery, 2012). Prototype robots have been developed to support independent living, in order to help older adults who try to live in their homes for as long as possible, even when the user is functionally disabled (Garcia-Soler *et al.*, 2018). The systems can help with daily living activities such as reaching, fetching

BOX 7.1 FACTORS INTEGRAL TO THE DEVELOPMENT AND OPERATIONALISATION OF INTEGRATED CARE

- Proactive approaches, building on the capabilities, assets and strengths of individuals and communities.
- Jurisdictional boundaries: complexity of governmental policy formulation, administration and regulation with respect to the provision of health and social care.
- Adequate investment and clarity on the funding mechanism: division and structure of funding for health and social care; universality vs means-tested; through pooled budgets, different organisations can contribute funds to a single entity, enabling a local authority and an NHS body to provide integrated health and social care services with shared outcomes.
- Local governance and management: legal and administrative relationships within and between stakeholders.
- National law, e.g. equality and non-discrimination under Equality Act 2010, and allowing for integration given s.75 of Health and Social Care Act 2012.
- Strategic planning: stakeholder involvement in joint planning and community needs assessment.
- Focus on continuity of care: consideration of, and alignment with, patient or user needs regardless of existing limitations in system, sector or setting (e.g. resources, eligibility).
- Ability to bundle and access a broad range of needed health and social care services from anywhere on the continuum of care.
- Ability to form networks or relationships: nature of working arrangements among and between institutions, providers and the wider community.
- Multidisciplinary approaches, team-working and leadership.
- Case finding: a legitimate ability to identify and target 'at-risk' populations. No screening when screening not justified.
- Commitment to performing comprehensive assessment, e.g. the CGA.
- Primary care: synchrony with general practitioners, other components of the primary care sector, as well as specialists.
- Case management and care planning: planning, arrangement and monitoring of needed care across time, place and discipline.
- Control over transitions between benefits, settings and providers.
- Teamwork: ongoing communication and collaboration among, and clinical management by, a multidisciplinary group of providers.
- Information-sharing: access to and use of shared information, e.g. electronic care or medical records within constraints of procedure on disclosure and confidentiality. Requires interoperability.
- System outcomes: overall responsibility for and evaluation of total quality, value and costs within budgetary constraints.
- Professional education and training, and workforce development.

Based on Kodner *et al.*, 2000, Box 1, p. 4.

and carrying objects that are heavy or out of reach (Pigini *et al.*, 2012). Alternatives in assistive technology options should all be fully considered. Telecare/AT options should be considered and optimised before a move to a care home.

As I introduced in the tail end of the previous chapter, frailty can affect a person's independence (Santos-Eggimann *et al.*, 2009) and is associated with institutionalisation (Rockwood *et al.*, 1996). The impetus for integration as a policy goal has been driven by three major factors. First, an ageing population and shifts in the pattern of disease means that more people are living longer with a mixture of needs – including complex comorbidity, frailty in very old age and dementia – that require coordinated care from different professionals, services and organisations. Often this requires long-term support closer to home rather than single episodes of care in acute hospitals (Humphries, 2015). Despite an increasing expectation that professionals and health and social care organisations should operate in an integrated way across organisational boundaries, there is a lack of understanding between care homes and the NHS about how the two sectors should work together (Gage *et al.*, 2012).

The annual incidence rate for disability, as represented in the long-term care insurance (LTCI) data, significantly decreased over time in the older population. Active life expectancy at age 70 years was substantially extended (Shinkai *et al.*, 2016). Multimorbid and/or frail patients may require services that are not frequently considered part of the clinical routine (e.g. support at home for activities of daily living, transportation, community care) but are crucial for the success of clinical interventions in this population. Interventions and treatments should be adopted, possibly following models of care of chronic diseases or multimorbidity (Onder *et al.*, 2017).

Urgent care

Frailty care needs to be tailored according to care settings, ranging from the emergency room to end of life.

It is worth noting Conroy and Turpin (2016, p. 584): 'Geriatricians are not numerous enough to deliver direct care to every frail older person, and it is not possible to place a geriatrician in every GP practice, nursing home, emergency department or acute medical unit all the time.' Hospitalised older people are often frail. Accurate identification of which patients are likely to encounter poor health outcomes is important for care planning and risk assessment for intended surgical or medical treatments (Ensrud *et al.*, 2009). Comans and colleagues (2016) found an increase of 22 and 43 per cent in the costs of six months of healthcare for a cohort of older people with intermediate and high levels of frailty compared with those with low frailty following a hospital admission. According to the NICE guideline:

> Health and social care practitioners should develop a care plan with adults who have identified social care needs and who are at risk of being admitted

to hospital. Include contingency planning for all aspects of the person's life. If they are admitted to hospital, refer to this plan.

('Transition between inpatient hospital settings and community or care home settings for adults with social care needs', page 5[11])

The 'critical time window' for interventions that target frailty has not yet been clearly established. On a spectrum from pre-frailty, to frailty, to disability, it is often assumed that early intervention to prevent the onset of disability is crucial and optimal; however, that is not to say that established disability cannot be reduced, or its progression slowed, or its impact on the older person and his or her caregivers mitigated (Cesari *et al.*, 2016). The course of disability in the last year of life did not follow a predictable pattern based on the condition leading to death (Gill *et al.*, 2010). The need for developing and implementing effective strategies aimed at delaying or preventing disability has been repeatedly underlined and is currently the main focus of several healthcare policies (Canevelli *et al.*, 2017). For more vulnerable patients it seems appropriate to move specialised hospital-based teams into the community, to minimise complications of prolonged hospitalisation and to manage complex conditions, to facilitate early community reintegration and to avoid institutionalisation (Mas *et al.*, 2016).

Palliative care, end of life and decision making

The principles of palliative care apply to any population that could benefit from a comprehensive, person-centred plan of care from the time of diagnosis through the entire illness trajectory (Raudonis and Daniel, 2010). Collaboration between geriatric and palliative care teams is of growing importance. Older adults are living longer and facing substantial symptoms related to malignant and non-malignant terminal illnesses (Grossman *et al.*, 2014). The end of life trajectory of the frail is well documented but identifying the start of a 'terminal phase' is challenging. This, coupled with the complex needs and high symptom burden of this group, makes it appropriate to introduce palliative care from diagnosis, with a naturally increasing emphasis on this approach as frailty advances (Pal and Manning, 2014). In a recent study, general practitioners demonstrated a strong commitment to caring for the frail older patients until the end of life. However, it is a challenging and complex task that requires significant time, which can take GPs to their limits. There is a great need to improve patient- and family-centred proactive communication, as well as inter-professional co-operation. Effective communication creates opportunities to identify goals and actions for supported self-care, and to build the necessary motivation and confidence to carry out the necessary changes. Strengthening the team approach in primary care could relieve the burden on GPs, especially in rural areas, while simultaneously improving end of life care for their patients (Geiger *et al.*, 2016).

The number of people in their last years of life with advanced chronic conditions, palliative care needs and limited life prognosis due to different causes, including multimorbidity, organ failure, frailty, dementia and cancer, is rising. Such people represent more than 1 per cent of the population. They are present in all care settings, cause around 75 per cent of mortalities, and may account for up to one-third of total national health system spend (Gómez-Batiste *et al.*, 2017). Understanding how best to provide palliative care for frail older people with non-malignant conditions is an international priority. Bone and colleagues (2016) aimed to develop a community-based episodic model of **short-term integrated palliative and supportive care** (SIPS) based on the views of service users and other key stakeholders in the United Kingdom. The SIPS model has been carefully developed in consultation with key stakeholders (Bone *et al.*, 2016). Exacerbations or episodes of decline are heterogeneous and unpredictable, leading to uncertainty about the indicators for referral to specialist palliative care (Murray *et al.*, 2005). Boockvar and Meier (2006) suggested palliative care (establishment of goals of care, symptom management, programmatic support, financial planning and family support) as appropriate at any stage of frailty.

Frail individuals are at high risk of losing their autonomy for everyday functioning (Ávila-Funes *et al.*, 2008). Also, frail individuals are acknowledged to be an optimal target population for the implementation of dependency prevention programmes (Cesari *et al.*, 2014). When to begin palliative care is a troublesome question for patients, families and healthcare providers. Older adults experience different markers for the initiation of palliative care than younger populations (Klick and Hauer, 2010). The following are disease-independent markers for beginning palliative care: frailty, functional dependence, cognitive impairment, symptom distress and family support needs (Morrison and Meir, 2003). Importantly, certain approaches, such as treatment of infections, or invasive investigations, can be included in advance care planning. It is especially important that **advance care planning** is not seen as a 'one-off event'; communication with patients and families is a continuous process and should be made available to patients with and without mental capacity, fully involving care partners/relatives in best interest decisions.

Family and care partners should be supported in considering options and making decisions. NICE offers clear guidance on **shared decision making**.[12] It is essential to recognise frail patients near the end of life, so discussions on goals of care, advance care directives and shared decision making, including early referrals to palliative and supportive care, can take place before an emergency arises (Cardona-Morrell *et al.*, 2017). According to the Health Foundation (2013, p. 6),[13] 'activated patients' are required to benefit fully from shared decision making. These are:

> Patients who are activated believe they have important roles to play in self-managing care, collaborating with providers, and maintaining their health; they know how to manage their condition and prevent health declines; and they have the skills and behavioural repertoire to manage their condition, collaborate with their health providers, maintain their health, and access appropriate and high quality care.

However, such interventions are likely to become clinically less beneficial, and potentially more harmful, as frailty progresses, with symptom control becoming an increasing focus towards the end of life. Encouraging people living with frailty to make decisions (for example, about treatment through 'activation') about their health is clearly important, but requires us to address the stigma which surrounds frailty.

> Communities can be harnessed to improve health and wellbeing and reduce health inequalities. Commissioning using an asset-based approach allows the NHS to access the wealth of experience and practical skills, knowledge, capacity and passion of local people, and to exploit the potential for communities to become equal partners in their care.
>
> *('Personalised care and support planning handbook: the journey to person-centred care: core Information', p. 19[14])*

Improved understanding of how to provide palliative care to the growing number of older people living with frailty, multimorbidity and nearing the end of life is an international priority. Care partners often organise community services (Productivity Commission, 2008), and are relied upon to enforce or encourage compliance to intervention strategies (Kaufman, 1994). Healthcare systems worldwide are struggling to deliver quality healthcare amidst challenges posed by ageing populations, the complexity of health states in old age and increasingly complex technology, which all have contributed to escalating costs (Lim *et al.*, 2017). It is noteworthy that the 'End of life care strategy' (Department of Health, 2008[15]) had been developed to build an integrated system to: provide care for frail elderly with advance illnesses, develop advance care programmes that respect patients' choices and promote high-quality end of life care. It is argued that frail older persons with cognitive impairment, who are in need of end of life care, should be deterred from unnecessary hospitalisation. The majority of these transfers to the emergency department can be avoided if there is better advance care planning beforehand, more specially trained nurses in elderly care and more home visits (Björck and Wijk, 2018).

The way in which primary care, especially GPs, engage with advance care planning (ACP), is very important for future service provision. 'Most GPs viewed ACP as important. However, their enthusiasm was tempered by experience. This study highlights the difficulties for GPs of encouraging dialogue and respecting individuals' wishes within the constraints of the existing health and social care system' (Sharp *et al.*, 2018).

A need to pursue resilience?

Whatever the care setting, there seems to be a wide degree of variation between individuals even towards death (Lloyd *et al.*, 2016). Stolz and colleagues (2017) found '**poverty risk**' associated with increased levels of frailty among older adults, and the gap persisted, even slightly increased throughout old age. Rather than educational or behavioural factors, material and, in particular, psychosocial factors, such as perceived control and social isolation, explained a large part of poverty risk-related differences in frailty. Recent results suggest that the overall slightly increasing birth-cohort trend in functional difficulties observed among current cohorts of older people in the UK hides underlying increases among low SES (socioeconomic status) individuals and a relative small reduction among high SES individuals. Further studies are needed to understand the causes of such trends and to propose appropriate interventions (Morciano et al., 2015). The framing of frailty, for example, through the accumulation of deficits and intrinsic capacity are very close, and complementary. They appear to be two sides of the same coin, and not in any way conflicting or contradictory. Frailty might be perceived as the age-related decline of physiological systems determining the reduction of intrinsic capacity, consequently leading to increased risk of negative health outcomes (Cesari, 2017). In response to the WHO's proactive approach to promoting intrinsic capacity through designing new systems for primary care for older persons living in the community, a step-care approach in early detection of problems and a guide to subsequent action, that allows for management in the community and reducing reliance on the hospital system, is being developed and piloted in Hong Kong (Woo et al., 2016).

There has been some interest in 'operationalising resilience'. A very useful review of various resilience measuring scales is provided by Windle et al. (2011) (see Box 7.2).

The significance of intrinsic capacity

Intrinsic capacity may also be seen as sharing some commonalities with the concept of resilience, but resilience is a concept that extends well beyond the biological status of the organism, and spreads over its social network, cultural background, economical capacities and living environment (Cesari et al., 2018).

> The focus on hospital-based, disease-based and self-contained 'silo' curative care models further undermines the ability of health systems to provide universal, equitable, high-quality and financially sustainable care. Service providers are often unaccountable to the populations they serve and therefore have limited incentive to provide the responsive care that matches the needs of their users. People are often unable to make appropriate decisions about their own health and health care, or exercise control over decisions about their health and that of their communities.
>
> (WHO, 2015, p. 9[16])

Although it is thought that genetic factors play a role in healthy ageing, the contribution is small compared with environmental factors. Studies into contributors of successful ageing highlighted healthy lifestyle (physical activity, nutrition),

---

BOX 7.2 OPERATIONALISING 'RESILIENCE'

The Connor–Davidson Resilience Scale (CD-RISC, Connor and Davidson, 2003) has been the prominent instrument for evaluating resilience with adequate psychometric properties. It comprises 25 items, each rated on a five-point scale (0–4), with higher scores reflecting greater resilience.

The Resilience Scale for Adults (RSA) was developed following inductive procedures: identification of protective factors in specialised literature, categorisation and empirical reduction of domains. The RSA evaluates four intrapersonal mechanisms of protection: confidence in abilities and judgments, and self-efficacy, the ability to plan ahead, being goal-oriented and having a positive outlook, the preference for having and following routines, and social warmth, flexibility and humour; as well as two social and family-oriented mechanisms of protection (Morote et al., 2017). The instrument developed by Friborg and colleagues (2003) is one of the few valid methods to evaluate adult protective mechanisms.

The Resilience Scale (RS), which measures the capacity to withstand life stressors, and to thrive and make meaning from challenges, consists of a 17-item 'Personal Competence' subscale and an 8-item 'Acceptance of Self and Life' subscale (Wagnild and Young, 1993).

The Baruth Protective Factors Inventory measures the construct of resilience by assessing four protective factors: adaptable personality, supportive environments, fewer stressors and compensating experiences (Baruth and Carroll 2002).

The Brief-Resilient Coping Scale measures the tendency to successfully adapt to and cope with stress. The purpose of this scale is to identify strong coping behaviours (Sinclair and Wallston 2004).

---

environmental enrichment and stress avoidance, and methods to preserve cognitive function by measures that promote neuronal plasticity (Woo et al., 2016). Current difficulties for ageing research include the inherent complexity of the changes that occur with age. The influence of the environment may be particularly strong in the event of natural or technological disasters and human–induced conflict. Yet although responses to these events typically prioritise assistance to vulnerable or marginalised groups, the needs of older adults are frequently overlooked (van Kessel et al., 2014). The focus of many studies on successful ageing has shifted from disease status and functional decline to multidimensional health status, which encompasses physical, functional, psychological and social health. Early published reports defined successful ageing using only one or two dimensions of health, such as the absence of chronic diseases, longer longevity, independent physical functioning, social life engagement and mental health (Li et al., 2014). Frailty is very common, with a prevalence in high-income countries at age 50–64 years of around 4 per cent, increasing to 17 per cent in people older than 65 years. In both high-resource and low-resource settings the prevalence of frailty is distributed along the socioeconomic gradient such that individuals with less education and income are more likely to be frail (Beard *et al.*, 2016).

Intrinsic capacity is defined by WHO as the combination of the individual's physical and mental (including psychosocial) capacities (World Health Organization, 2015). Functional ability, in contrast, relates to the combination and interaction of an individual's intrinsic capacity, and the characteristics of the environment he or she inhabits. A shift in the type of care older people receive is also needed: away from a singular focus on the management of specific diseases and conditions and towards care that aims to optimise older people's intrinsic capacity over their life course (Ham, 2010; Low *et al.*, 2011; Eklund and Wilhelmson, 2009). The size of the population of older persons who may have lost much of their intrinsic capacity can be reduced, it is argued, substantially through health policies.

But the problem remains as to how *exactly* do you operationalise the 'index of intrinsic capacity'. Using the **International Classification of Functioning, Disability and Health**[17] framework as background and taking into account available evidence, five domains (i.e. locomotion, vitality, cognition, psychological, sensory) are identified as pivotal for capturing the individual's intrinsic capacity (and therefore also reserves) and, through this, pave the way for its objective measurement (Cesari *et al.*, 2018). The evolution of assets, deficits and resilience across the whole of the life course appears to be pivotal.

Take for example, Bektas and colleagues' (2017, p. 10) following comment: 'Longitudinal studies with a life course approach are needed to gain further mechanistic insight on the processes that lead to functional decline with ageing, and the role played in this process by inflammation and environmental challenges.' Operationalising intrinsic capacity will be very important. In 1999, Stuck and colleagues had conducted a systematic review of the literature aimed at measuring the strength of evidence linking different risk factors to functional decline in older persons. In particular, Stuck and colleagues identified impairments in mood (i.e. depressive symptoms), sociality (i.e. participation in social activities), cognition, physical performance, homeostatic balance (i.e. weight loss, abnormal body mass index) and vision (i.e. reduced visual acuity) as strong predictors of care dependence.

To meet the challenges of ageing populations, WHO has advocated healthy ageing as a goal, with an emphasis on function or maintaining/promoting intrinsic capacity. This requires reorientation of health policy and systems to shift to integrated care of older people in the community from specialty dominated hospital care, as well as regular activities in the community, to adopt and maintain a lifestyle to reduce frailty and disability (or promote intrinsic capacity). Redesigning a responsive health system requires a top-down approach with financial incentives to service providers, the development of information systems collecting data for intrinsic capacity (or frailty), as well as training for the health and social care workforce in care of older people (Woo, 2017). It is, however, entirely possible that all of a solution is still provided by a medical model.

According to WHO, a comprehensive public health action on population ageing is urgently needed. This will require fundamental shifts in how we think about ageing itself. WHO's *World report on ageing and health* (p. vii)[18] outlines a framework for action to foster 'Healthy ageing' built around the new concepts of functional ability and intrinsic capacity.

> The resulting diversity in the capacities and health needs of older people is not random, but rooted in events throughout the life course that can often be modified, underscoring the importance of a life-course approach. Though most older people will eventually experience multiple health problems, older age does not imply dependence. Moreover, contrary to common assumptions, ageing has far less influence on health care expenditures than other factors, including the high costs of new medical technologies.

This will require a transformation of health systems away from disease-based curative models and towards the provision of older-person-centred and integrated care.

I return, however, to a central pervasive theme throughout this book. **Resilience** is a nascent concept that can be understood in various ways when viewed through the lens of differing disciplines, and has been an enduring pervasive theme of this entire book. Resilience can be used in a strengths-based approach within a public health framework to enhance the proportion of the population that experiences efficient recovery. Resilience can be understood as 'the intrinsic capacity of a system, community or society predisposed to a shock or stress to adapt and survive by changing its non-essential attributes and rebuilding itself' (Manyena, 2006, p. 446). The resilience concept can be observed in a number of documents, such as the Hyogo Framework for Action 2005–2015, which is the International Strategy for Disaster Reduction and aims to build the resilience of nations and communities to disasters (United Nations, 2007).

> There is also a lack of consensus on what constitutes a positive outcome for older people. Traditionally, health-care research has used indicators of disease, disability, longevity, patient and provider satisfaction, health-care utilization, hospitalization, institutionalization and cost. In contrast, the main aim of integrated care for older people is not to manage disease or prolong life but is, instead, to optimize older people's intrinsic capacity over their life course and, hence, ensure healthy ageing.
>
> *(Araujo de Carvalho et al., 2017, p. 760[19])*

Overall, it will be essential to put resilience or intrinsic capacity, as well as assets and deficits, at the heart of future debates on frailty. Overall, there are currently a number of key gaps in our understanding of this area (see Table 7.1). Leadership is essential in delivering compassionate person-centred care, and overall team practices should champion diversity, equality and inclusion.

TABLE 7.1 Current gaps and opportunities in training and practice areas for frailty

Training and practice area	Potential gap	Opportunities for enhanced leadership and skill development
Education and training	Professionals and practitioners may enter practice without knowing how to measure frailty or interpret specific findings of frailty instruments. Clinical and research networks are seeking out gaps, issues or areas in training and education you feel could be met or supported, and looking for any relevant links, resources or information on existing frailty education. Diverse methods of frailty measurement and operationalisation have roots in differing conceptual views regarding its definition.	Provide training in frailty recognition to all health and social care staff who are likely to encounter older people. For example, the 'National Frailty Education Programme' philosophy is based on the belief that education increases knowledge and enhances healthcare professionals' skills in clinical areas (https://britishgeriatricssociety.wordpress.com/2018/02/05/can-a-national-frailty-education-programme-be-a-driver-of-culture-change-in-healthcare). See also 'Frailty Core Capabilities Framework' (www.skillsforhealth.org.uk/services/item/607-frailty-core-capabilities-framework).
Practice guidelines/ evidence	For example: BGS: Fit for frailty NIHR: Comprehensive care	Need to be continually updated
Proactive care team leadership	The need for interdisciplinary leadership and strategic membership of teams, including allied health professionals, is anticipated	Critical to find ways to optimise proactive care by personalised care and support planning Needs 'buy in' from clinical leaders and managers
Health and social care outcomes; audit, service improvement and research	The past decade has already seen a significant increase in the number of peer-reviewed publications on frailty	Engage in/publish clinical and health outcomes research on frailty

Notes

1 http://clahrc-cp.nihr.ac.uk/wp-content/uploads/2012/07/Evaluation_GUIDE.pdf, p. 8.
2 www.nuffieldtrust.org.uk/files/2017-01/evaluating-integrated-community-care-web-final.pdf.
3 www.northumberlandccg.nhs.uk/wp-content/uploads/2013/09/FEPP-Judging-Panel-Presentation-3-2.pdf.

4 www.england.nhs.uk/wp-content/uploads/2014/02/safe-comp-care.pdf.
5 www.england.nhs.uk/blog/martin-mcshane-23.
6 http://learning.wm.hee.nhs.uk/sites/default/files/ICT_Care%20Navigation%20Competency%20Framework.pdf.
7 www.who.int/disabilities/care/NeedToScaleUpRehab.pdf?ua1.
8 Clegg A, Clarke D, Cundill B, Farrin A, Forster A, Goodwin V, Hartley S, Hulme C, Wright P, Young J. *RCT evaluation of a home-based exercise intervention as extended rehabilitation for older people with frailty after discharge from hospital or intermediate care.* NIHR HTA. £2 million (March 2017 to June 2021).
9 www.who.int/servicedeliverysafety/areas/people-centred-care/framework/en.
10 www.kingsfund.org.uk/sites/default/files/field/field_publication_file/policy-framework-integrated-care-older-people-developed-carmen-network-penny-banks-1-august-2004.pdf.
11 1 December 2015, www.nice.org.uk/guidance/ng27.
12 www.nice.org.uk/about/what-we-do/our-programmes/nice-guidance/nice-guidelines/shared-decision-making.
13 Health Foundation, April 2013, *Implementing shared decision making*, www.health.org.uk/sites/health/files/ImplementingSharedDecisionMaking.pdf.
14 www.england.nhs.uk/wp-content/uploads/2016/04/core-info-care-support-planning-1.pdf.
15 www.cpa.org.uk/cpa/End_of_Life_Care_Strategy.pdf.
16 http://apps.who.int/gb/ebwha/pdf_files/WHA69/A69_39-en.pdf.
17 www.who.int/classifications/icf/en.
18 http://apps.who.int/iris/bitstream/10665/186463/1/9789240694811_eng.pdf.
19 www.who.int/bulletin/volumes/95/11/16-187617/en.

References

Araujo de Carvalho I, Epping-Jordan J, Pot AM, Kelley E, Toro N, Thiyagarajan JA, Beard JR. (2017). Organizing integrated health-care services to meet older people's needs. *Bull World Health Organ.* November 1; 95(11): 756–63. doi:10.2471/BLT.16.187617. Epub 2017 May 26.

Ávila-Funes JA, Helmer C, Amieva H, Barberger-Gateau P, Le Goff M, Ritchie K *et al.* (2008). Frailty among community-dwelling elderly people in France: the three-city study. *J Gerontol Ser A Biol Sci Med Sci.* 63: 1089–96. doi:10.1093/gerona/63.10.1089.

Baruth KE, Carroll JJ. (2002). A formal assessment of resilience: The Baruth Protective Factors Inventory. *Journal of Individual Psychology.* 58: 235–44.

Beard JR, Bloom DE. (2015). Towards a comprehensive public health response to population ageing. *Lancet.* February 14; 385(9968): 658–61. doi:10.1016/S0140-6736(14)61461-6. Epub 2014 November 6.

Beard JR, Officer A, de Carvalho IA, Sadana R, Pot AM, Michel JP, Lloyd-Sherlock P, Epping Jordan JE, Peeters GMEEG, Mahanani WR, Thiyagarajan JA, Chatterji S. (2016). The World report on ageing and health: a policy framework for healthy ageing. *Lancet.* May 21; 387(10033): 2145–54. doi:10.1016/S0140-6736(15)00516-4. Epub 2015 October 29.

Bektas A, Schurman SH, Sen R, Ferrucci L. (2017). Aging, inflammation and the environment. *Exp Gerontol.* December 21. pii: S0531–5565(17)30779–9. doi:10.1016/j.exger.2017.12.015. [Epub ahead of print].

Béland F, Hollander MJ. (2011). Integrated models of care delivery for the frail elderly: international perspectives. *Gac Sanit.* December; 25(Suppl. 2): 138–46. doi:10.1016/j.gaceta.2011.09.003. Epub 2011 November 15.

Björck M, Wijk H. (2018). Is hospitalisation necessary? A survey of frail older persons with cognitive impairment transferred from nursing homes to the emergency department. *Scand J Caring Sci*. February 12. doi:10.1111/scs.12559. [Epub ahead of print].

Bone AE, Morgan M, Maddocks M, Sleeman KE, Wright J, Taherzadeh S, Ellis-Smith C, Higginson IJ, Evans CJ. (2016). Developing a model of short-term integrated palliative and supportive care for frail older people in community settings: perspectives of older people, care partners and other key stakeholders. *Age Ageing*. November; 45(6): 863–73. Epub 2016 September 1.

Boockvar KS, Meier DE. (2006). Palliative care for frail older adults. *JAMA*. 296: 2245–53.

Borgstrom E. (2017). Social Death. *QJM*. January; 110(1): 5–7. doi:10.1093/qjmed/hcw183. Epub 2016 October 20.

Calciolari S, Ilinca S. (2016). Unraveling care integration: assessing its dimensions and antecedents in the Italian Health System. *Health Policy*. January; 120(1): 129–38. doi:10.1016/j.healthpol.2015.12.002. Epub 2015 December 13.

Canevelli M, Bruno G, Remiddi F, Vico C, Lacorte E, Vanacore N, Cesari M. (2017). Spontaneous reversion of clinical conditions measuring the risk profile of the individual: from frailty to mild cognitive impairment. *Front Med* (Lausanne). October 30; 4: 184. doi:10.3389/fmed.2017.00184. eCollection 2017.

Cardona-Morrell M, Lewis E, Suman S, Haywood C, Williams M, Brousseau AA, Greenaway S, Hillman K, Dent E. (2017). Recognising older frail patients near the end of life: What next? *Eur J Intern Med*. November; 45: 84–90. doi:10.1016/j.ejim.2017.09.026. Epub 2017 October 6.

Cesari, M. (2017). Intersections between frailty and the concept of intrinsic capacity. *Innovation in Aging*. 1(Suppl. 1): 692. doi:10.1093/geroni/igx004.2479.

Cesari M, Araujo De Carvalho I, Amuthavalli Thiyagarajan J, Cooper C, Finbarr M, Register J-Y, Vellas B, Beard J. (2018). Evidence for the domains supporting the construct for intrinsic capacity. *J Gerontol A Biol Sci Med Sci*. February 2. doi:10.1093/gerona/gly011. [Epub ahead of print].

Cesari M, Gambassi G, van Kan GA, Vellas B. (2014). The frailty phenotype and the frailty index: different instruments for different purposes. *Age Ageing*. 43: 10–12. doi:10.1093/ageing/aft160.

Cesari M, Prince M, Thiyagarajan JA, De Carvalho IA, Bernabei R, Chan P, Gutierrez-Robledo LM, Michel JP, Morley JE, Ong P, Rodriguez Manas L, Sinclair A, Won CW, Beard J, Vellas B. (2016). Frailty: an emerging public health priority. *J Am Med Dir Assoc*. March 1; 17(3): 188–92. doi:10.1016/j.jamda.2015.12.016. Epub 2016 January 21.

Christensen K, Doblhammer G, Rau R, Vaupel JW. (2009). Ageing populations: the challenges ahead. *Lancet*. 374(9696): 1196–208. doi:10.1016/S0140 6736(09)61460-4.

Clegg A, Young J, Iliffe S, Rikkert M, Rockwood K. (2013). Frailty in elderly people. *Lancet*. 381(9868): 752–62. doi:10.1016/S0140-6736(12)62167-9.

Cohen-Mansfield J, Skornick-Bouchbinder M, Brill S. (2017). Trajectories of end of life: a systematic review. *J Gerontol B Psychol Sci Soc Sci*. July 8. doi:10.1093/geronb/gbx093. [Epub ahead of print].

Comans TA, Peel NM, Hubbard RE, Mulligan AD, Gray LC, Scuffham PA. (2016). The increase in healthcare costs associated with frailty in older people discharged to a post-acute transition care program. *Age Ageing*. March; 45(2): 317–20. doi:10.1093/ageing/afv196. Epub 2016 January 13.

Connor KM, Davidson JR. (2003). Development of a new resilience scale: the Connor-Davidson Resilience Scale (CD-RISC). *Depression and Anxiety*. 18: 76–82. doi:10.1002/da.10113.

Conroy S, Dowsing T. (2013). The ability of frailty to predict outcomes in older people attending an acute medical unit. *Acute Med*. 12: 74–6.

Conroy SP, Turpin S. (2016). New horizons: urgent care for older people with frailty. *Age Ageing.* September; 45(5): 577–84. doi:10.1093/ageing/afw135. Epub 2016 August 1.

Covinsky KE, Eng C, Lui LY, Sands LP, Yaffe K. (2003). The last 2 years of life: functional trajectories of frail older people. *J Am Geriatr Soc.* April; 51(4): 492–8.

Dannefer D. (2003). Cumulative advantage and the life course. *J Gerontology.* 58(b): 327–37.

de Bruin SR, Versnel N, Lemmens LC, Molema CC, Schellevis FG, Nijpels G, Baan CA. (2012). Comprehensive care programs for patients with multiple chronic conditions: a systematic literature review. *Health Policy.* October; 107(2–3): 108–45. doi:10.1016/j.healthpol.2012.06.006. Epub 2012 August 9.

Dubuc N, Bonin L, Tourigny A, Mathieu L, Couturier Y, Tousignant M, Corbin C, Delli-Colli N, Raîche M. (2013). Development of integrated care pathways: toward a care management system to meet the needs of frail and disabled community-dwelling older people. *Int J Integr Care.* May 17; 13: e017. Print 2013 April.

Eklund K, Wilhelmson K. (2009). Outcomes of coordinated and integrated interventions targeting frail elderly people: a systematic review of randomised controlled trials. *Health Soc Care Community.* September; 17(5): 447–58. doi:10.1111/j.1365-2524.2009.00844.x. pmid: 19245421.

Elliott A, Hull L, Conroy SP. (2017). Frailty identification in the emergency department: a systematic review focussing on feasibility. *Age Ageing.* May 1; 46(3): 509–513. doi:10.1093/ageing/afx019.

Ensrud KE, Ewing SK, Cawthon PM, Fink HA, Taylor BC, Cauley JA. (2009). A comparison of frailty indexes for the prediction of falls, disability, fractures, and mortality in older men. *J Am Geriatr Soc.* 57: 492–8.

Espinoza S, Walston JD. (2005). Frailty in older adults: insights and interventions. *Cleveland Clinic Journal of Medicine.* 72(12): 1105–12.

Fabbricotti IN, Janse B, Looman WM, de Kuijper R, van Wijngaarden JD, Reiffers A. (2013). Integrated care for frail elderly compared to usual care: a study protocol of a quasi-experiment on the effects on the frail elderly, their caregivers, health professionals and health care costs. *BMC Geriatr.* April 12; 13: 31. doi:10.1186/1471-2318-13-31.

Friborg O, Hjemdal O, Rosenvinge JH, Martinussen M. (2003). A new rating scale for adult resilience: what are the central protective resources behind healthy adjustment? *Int J Methods Psychiatr Res.* 12(2): 65–76.

Gage H, Dickinson A, Victor C, Williams P, Cheynel J, Davies SL, Iliffe S, Froggatt K, Martin W, Goodman C. (2012). Integrated working between residential care homes and primary care: a survey of care homes in England. *BMC Geriatr.* November 14; 12: 71. doi:10.1186/1471-2318-12-71.

García-Soler Á, Facal D, Díaz-Orueta U, Pigini L, Blasi L, Qiu R. (2018). Inclusion of service robots in the daily lives of frail older users: a step-by-step definition procedure on users' requirements. *Arch Gerontol Geriatr.* January; 74: 191–6. doi:10.1016/j.archger.2017.10.024. Epub 2017 October 31.

Geiger K, Schneider N, Bleidorn J, Klindtworth K, Jünger S, Müller-Mundt G. (2016). Caring for frail older people in the last phase of life: the general practitioners' view. *BMC Palliat Care.* June 2; 15: 52. doi:10.1186/s12904-016-0124-5.

Gill TM, Gahbauer EA, Han L, Allore HG. (2010). Trajectories of disability in the last year of life. *N Engl J Med.* April 1; 362(13): 1173–80. doi:10.1056/NEJMoa0909087.

Gómez-Batiste X, Murray S, Thomas K, Blay C, Boyd K, Moine S, Gignon M, den Eynden BV, Leysen B, Wens J, Engels Y, Dees M, Costantini M. (2017). Comprehensive and integrated palliative care for people with advanced chronic conditions: an update from several European initiatives and recommendations for policy. *Journal of Pain and Symptom Management.* doi:10.1016/j.jpainsymman.2016.10.361.

Grossman D, Rootenberg M, Perri GA, Yogaparan T, DeLeon M, Calabrese S, Grief CJ, Moore J, Gill A, Stilos K, Daines P, Zimmermann C, Mazzotta P. (2014). Enhancing communication in end-of-life care: a clinical tool translating between the Clinical Frailty Scale and the Palliative Performance Scale. *J Am Geriatr Soc*. August; 62(8): 1562–7. doi:10.1111/jgs.12926. Epub 2014 June 24.

Gwyther H, Shaw R, Jaime Dauden E-A, D'Avanzo B, Kurpas D, Bujnowska-Fedak M *et al*. (2018). Understanding frailty: a qualitative study of European healthcare policymakers' approaches to frailty screening and management. *BMJ Open*. 8: e018653. doi:10.1136/bmjopen-2017-018653.

Ham C. (2010). The ten characteristics of the high-performing chronic care system. *Health Econ Policy Law*. January; 5(Pt 1): 71–90.

Health Foundation. (2013). *Improving the flow of older people: Sheffield Teaching Hospital NHS Trust's experience of the Flow Cost Quality improvement programme*. www.health.org.uk/publication/improving-patient-flow.

Holroyd-Leduc J, Resin J, Ashley L, Barwich D, Elliott J, Huras P, Légaré F, Mahoney M, Maybee A, McNeil H, Pullman D, Sawatzky R, Stolee P, Muscedere J. (2016). Giving voice to older adults living with frailty and their family caregivers: engagement of older adults living with frailty in research, health care decision making, and in health policy. *Res Involv Engagem*. June 17; 2: 23. doi:10.1186/s40900-016-0038-7. eCollection 2016.

Humphries R. (2015). Integrated health and social care in England: progress and prospects. *Health Policy*. July; 119(7): 856–9. doi:10.1016/j.healthpol.2015.04.010. Epub 2015 May 6.

Karunananthan S, Wolfson C, Bergman H, Béland F, Hogan D. (2009). A multidisciplinary systematic literature review on frailty: overview of the methodology used by the Canadian Initiative on Frailty and Aging. *BMC Medical Research Methodology*. 9(68): 1–11. doi:10.1186/1471-2288-9-68.

Kaufman SR. (1994). The social construction of frailty: an anthropological perspective. *J Aging Stud*. 8: 45–58.

Klick JC, Hauer J. (2010). Pediatric palliative care. *Curr Probl Pediatr Adolesc Health Care*. July; 40(6): 120–51. doi:10.1016/j.cppeds.2010.05.001.

Kodner DL, Kyriacou CK. (2000). Fully integrated care for frail elderly: two American models. *Int J Integr Care*. November 1; 1: e08.

Kojima G, Iliffe S, Taniguchi Y, Shimada H, Rakugi H, Walters K. (2017). Prevalence of frailty in Japan: a systematic review and meta-analysis. *J Epidemiol*. August; 27(8): 347–53. doi:10.1016/j.je.2016.09.008. Epub 2016 November 15.

Koller K, Rockwood K. (2013). Frailty in older adults: implications for end-of-life care. *Cleve Clin J Med*. March; 80(3): 168–74. doi:10.3949/ccjm.80a.12100.

Li CI, Lin CH, Lin WY, Liu CS, Chang CK, Meng NH, Lee YD, Li TC1, Lin CC. (2014). Successful aging defined by health-related quality of life and its determinants in community-dwelling elders. *BMC Public Health*. September 28; 14: 1013. doi:10.1186/1471-2458-14-1013.

Lim WS, Wong SF, Leong I, Choo P, Pang WS. (2017). Forging a frailty-ready healthcare system to meet population ageing. *Int J Environ Res Public Health*. November 24; 14(12). pii: E1448. doi:10.3390/ijerph14121448.

Lloyd A, Kendall M, Starr JM, Murray SA. (2016). Physical, social, psychological and existential trajectories of loss and adaptation towards the end of life for older people living with frailty: a serial interview study. *BMC Geriatr*. October 20; 16(1): 176.

Looman WM, Fabbricotti IN, de Kuyper R, Huijsman R. (2016). The effects of a proactive integrated care intervention for frail community-dwelling older people: a quasi-experimental study with the GP-practice as single entry point. *BMC Geriatr*. February 15; 16: 43. doi:10.1186/s12877 016-0214-5.

Low LF, Yap M, Brodaty H. (2011). A systematic review of different models of home and community care services for older persons. *BMC Health Serv Res.* May 9; 11(1): 93. doi:10.1186/1472-6963-11-93MPMID:21549010.

Lyratzopoulos G, Elliott MN, Barbiere JM, Staetsky L, Paddison CA, Campbell J, Roland M. (2011). How can health care organizations be reliably compared? Lessons from a national survey of patient experience. *Med Care.* August; 49(8): 724–33. doi:10.1097/MLR.0b013e31821b3482.

Manyena SB. (2006). The concept of resilience revisited. *Disasters.* December; 30(4): 433–50.

Mas MÀ, Closa C, Santaeugènia SJ, Inzitari M, Ribera A, Gallofré M. (2016). Hospital-at-home integrated care programme for older patients with orthopaedic conditions: early community reintegration maximising physical function. *Maturitas.* June; 88: 65–9. doi:10.1016/j.maturitas.2016.03.005. Epub 2016 March 11.

McKeown J, Clarke A, Repper J. (2006). Life story work in health and social care: systematic literature review. *J Adv Nurs.* July; 55(2): 237–47.

Moorhouse P, Mallery LH. (2012). Palliative and therapeutic harmonization: a model for appropriate decision-making in frail older adults. *J Am Geriatr Soc.* December; 60(12): 2326–32. doi:10.1111/j.1532-5415.2012.04210.x. Epub 2012 October 30.

Morciano M, Hancock RM, Pudney SE. (2015). Birth-cohort trends in older-age functional disability and their relationship with socio-economic status: evidence from a pooling of repeated cross sectional population-based studies for the UK. *Soc Sci Med.* July; 136–7: 1–9. doi:10.1016/j.socscimed.2015.04.035. Epub 2015 May 6.

Morote R, Hjemdal O, Krysinska K, Martinez Uribe P, Corveleyn J. (2017). Resilience or hope? Incremental and convergent validity of the resilience scale for adults (RSA) and the Herth hope scale (HHS) in the prediction of anxiety and depression. *BMC Psychol.* October 27; 5(1): 36. doi:10.1186/s40359-017-0205-0.

Morrison RS, Meir DE (eds). (2003). *Geriatric palliative care.* New York: Oxford University Press.

Murray SA, Kendall M, Boyd K, Sheikh A. (2005). Illness trajectories and palliative care. *BMJ.* April 30; 330(7498): 1007–11.

NHS England. (2014). *Safe, compassionate care for frail older people using an integrated care pathway: practical guidance for commissioners, providers and nursing, medical and allied health professional leaders.* www.england.nhs.uk/wp-content/uploads/2014/02/safe-comp-care.pdf.

NIHR Dissemination Centre. (2017). *Themed review. Comprehensive care: older people living with frailty in hospitals.* www.dc.nihr.ac.uk/themed-reviews/Comprehensive-Care-final.pdf.

Onder G, Cesari M, Maggio M, Palmer K. (2017). Defining a care pathway for patients with multimorbidity or frailty. *Eur J Intern Med.* March; 38: 1–2. doi:10.1016/j.ejim.2017.01.013. Epub 2017 January 19.

Pal LM, Manning L. (2014). Palliative care for frail older people. *Clin Med* (Lond). June; 14(3): 292–5. doi:10.7861/clinmedicine.14-3-292.

Pigini L, Facal D, Garcia A, Burmester M, Andrich R. (2012). The proof of concept of a shadow robotic system for independent living at home. In: Miesenberger A, Penaz P, Zagler W (eds), *Computers helping people with special needs,* Vol. 7382. Berlin: Heide, pp. 634–41.

Productivity Commission. (2008). *Trends in aged care services: some implications.* Canberra.

Raudonis BM, Daniel K. (2010). Frailty: an indication for palliative care. *Geriatr Nurs.* September–October; 31(5): 379–84.

Rockwood K, Stolee P, McDowell I. (1996). Factors associated with institutionalization of older people in Canada: testing a multifactorial definition of frailty. *J Am Geriatr Soc.* May; 44(5): 578–82.

Santos-Eggimann B, Cuénoud P, Spagnoli J, Junod J. (2009). Prevalence of frailty in middle-aged and older community-dwelling Europeans living in 10 countries. *J Gerontol A Biol Sci Med Sci.* June; 64(6): 675–81. doi:10.1093/gerona/glp012. Epub 2009 March 10.

Senior HE, Parsons M, Kerse N, Chen MH, Jacobs S, Hoorn SV, Anderson CS. (2014). Promoting independence in frail older people: a randomised controlled trial of a restorative care service in New Zealand. *Age Ageing.* May; 43(3): 418–24. doi:10.1093/ageing/afu025. Epub 2014 March 4.

Sharp T, Malyon A, Barclay S. (2018). GPs' perceptions of advance care planning with frail and older people: a qualitative study. *Br J Gen Pract.* January; 68(666): 44–53. doi:10.3399/bjgp17X694145. Epub 2017 December 18.

Shinkai S, Yoshida H, Taniguchi Y, Murayama H, Nishi M, Amano H, Nofuji Y, Seino S, Fujiwara Y. (2016). Public health approach to preventing frailty in the community and its effect on healthy aging in Japan. *Geriatr Gerontol Int.* March; 16(Suppl. 1): 87–97. doi:10.1111/ggi.12726.

Silvester KM, Mohammed MA, Harriman P, Girolami A, Downes TW. (2014). Timely care for frail older people referred to hospital improves efficiency and reduces mortality without the need for extra resources. *Age Ageing.* July; 43(4): 472–7. doi:10.1093/ageing/aft170. Epub 2013 November 12.

Sinclair VG, Wallston KA. (2004). The development and psychometric evaluation of the Brief Resilient Coping Scale. *Assessment.* 11: 94–101.

Soong J, Poots AJ, Scott S, Donald K, Woodcock T, Lovett D, Bell D. (2015). Quantifying the prevalence of frailty in English hospitals. *BMJ Open.* October 21; 5(10): e008456. doi:10.1136/bmjopen 2015-008456.

Spoorenberg SLW, Uittenbroek RJ, Mindell B, Kremer BPH, Reijneveld SA, Wynial K. (2013). Embrace, a model for integrated elderly care: study protocol of a randomized controlled trial on the effectiveness regarding patient outcomes, service use, costs, and quality of care. *BMC Geriatrics.* 13: 62.

Stolz E, Mayerl H, Waxenegger A, Freidl W. (2017). Explaining the impact of poverty on old-age frailty in Europe: material, psychosocial and behavioural factors. *Eur J Public Health.* May 31. doi:10.1093/eurpub/ckx079. [Epub ahead of print].

Thwaites R, Glasby J, le Mesurier N, Littlechild R. (2017). Room for one more? A review of the literature on 'inappropriate' admissions to hospital for older people in the English NHS. *Health Soc Care Community.* January; 25(1): 1–10. doi:10.1111/hsc.12281. Epub 2015 October 5.

Turner G, Clegg A. British Geriatrics Society; Age UK; Royal College of General Practioners. (2014). Best practice guidelines for the management of frailty: a British Geriatrics Society, Age UK and Royal College of General Practitioners report. *Age Ageing.* November; 43(6): 744–7. doi:10.1093/ageing/afu138.

Uittenbroek RJ, Reijneveld SA, Stewart RE, Spoorenberg SL, Kremer HP, Wynia K. (2016). Development and psychometric evaluation of a measure to evaluate the quality of integrated care: the Patient Assessment of Integrated Elderly Care. *Health Expect.* August; 19(4): 962–72. doi:10.1111/hex.12391. Epub 2015 July 31.

United Nations. (2007). *Hyogo Framework for Action 2005–2015: Building the resilience of nations and communities to disasters.* United Nations Office for Disaster Risk Reduction, The International Strategy for Disaster Reduction.

van Kessel G, MacDougall C, Gibbs L. (2014). Resilience – rhetoric to reality: a systematic review of intervention studies after disasters. *Disaster Med Public Health Prep.* October; 8(5): 452–60. doi:10.1017/dmp. 2014.104. Epub 2014 October 24.

Wagnild GM, Young HM. (1993). Development and psychometric evaluation of the Resilience Scale. *J Nurs Meas.* Winter; 1(2): 165–78.

Walker A. (2006). Re-examining the political economy of ageing. In: Baars J, Dannefer D, Phillipson C, Walker A (eds), *Ageing, globalisation and inequality*. New York: Baywood, pp. 59–80.

Walsh B, Addington-Hall J, Roberts HC, Nicholls PG, Corner J. (2012). Outcomes after unplanned admission to hospital in older people: ill-defined conditions as potential indicators of the frailty trajectory. *J Am Geriatr Soc*. November; 60(11): 2104–9. doi:10.1111/j.1532 5415.2012.04198.x. Epub 2012 October 5.

Windle G, Bennett KM, Noyes J. (2011). A methodological review of resilience measurement scales. *Health Qual Life Outcomes*. February 4; 9: 8. doi:10.1186/1477-7525-9-8.

Woo J. (2017). Designing fit-for-purpose health and social services for ageing populations. *Int J Environ Res Public Health*. April 25; 14(5). pii: E457. doi:10.3390/ijerph14050457.

Woo J, Leung J, Zhang T. (2016). Successful aging and frailty: opposite sides of the same coin? *J Am Med Dir Assoc*. September 1; 17(9): 797–801. doi:10.1016/j.jamda.2016.04.015. Epub 2016 May 25.

World Health Organization. (2015). Summary. *World report on ageing and health*. http://apps.who.int/iris/bitstream/10665/186468/1/WHO_FWC_ALC_15.01_eng.pdf.

World Health Organization Europe. (2010). *Environment and health risks: a review of the influence and effects of social inequalities*. www.euro.who.int/__data/assets/pdf_file/0003/78069/E93670.pdf.

AFTERWORD

Introduction

There is indeed much to be excited about in the field of frailty. Frailty is clearly at the pivot of clinical care, and more resources and care should be made available to people who are frail – not less. Primary care commissioners should ensure that the needs of frail older people are at the heart of their commissioning. Older people with frailty are amongst the most in need of medical and social care continuity, and will have significant medical requirements.

Older people living with frailty can present to hospital with atypical symptoms and complex needs (NIHR Dissemination Centre, 2017). The current future direction, and indeed past, of 'frailty', for both service provision and research at least, are both intimately linked with the angle of perspective you decide to choose. *Anekāntavāda* (Sanskrit: अनेकान्तवाद., 'many-sidedness') refers to the Jain doctrine about metaphysical truths that emerged in ancient India; it states that the 'ultimate truth and reality' is complex, has multiple aspects.[1]

The Jain texts explain the *anekāntvāda* concept using the parable of blind men and elephant, in a manner similar to those found in both Buddhist and Hindu texts about limits of perception and the importance of complete context.

A famous parable has several Indian variations, but broadly goes as follows:

> A group of blind men heard that a strange animal, called an elephant, had been brought to the town, but none of them were aware of its shape and form. They then tried to deduce its form from some preliminary investigations. In the case of the first person, whose hand landed on the trunk, he said 'This being is like a thick snake'. For another one whose hand reached its ear, it seemed like a kind of fan. As for another person, whose hand was upon its leg, he said, the elephant is a pillar like a tree-trunk. The blind man who placed his hand upon its side said, 'The elephant is a wall' …[2]

The 'ultimate truth and reality' in frailty are sometimes difficult to see, when processes, procedures and policies appear to be so dominant in the discourse. That's the beauty of the 'frailty elephant'.

Further thoughts on identifying frailty

Part of the drive to wanting to 'do something' about frailty, as for dementia, is that there appears to be so much at stake in terms of exposure to the risk of increased morbidity and mortality. As for dementia, the rationale has been to hope to intervene in a more timely way, with more accurate timely diagnoses. Frailty could learn lessons here from other fields such as dementia.

Artificial intelligence (AI) is a field of computer science that aims to mimic human thought processes, learning capacity and knowledge storage. AI techniques have been applied, for example, in cardiovascular medicine to explore novel genotypes and phenotypes in existing diseases, improve the quality of patient care, enable cost-effectiveness, and reduce readmission and mortality rates (Krittanawong *et al.*, 2017). Precision medicine is a new paradigm that combines diagnostic, imaging and analytical tools to produce accurate diagnoses and therapeutic interventions tailored to the individual patient. This approach stands in contrast to the traditional 'one size fits all' concept, according to which researchers develop disease treatments and preventions for an 'average' patient without considering individual differences.

Key contributors to the heterogeneity found within frailty are that individuals belong to a range of disease subtypes (giving rise to **phenotypic heterogeneity**) and are at different stages of a dynamic disease process (producing **temporal heterogeneity**). If frailty is viewed as a number of different symptom clusters, involving heterogeneity, a 'swiss army knife' approach to managing frailty might, in fact, reap dividends. The 'one size fits all' concept has led to many ineffective or inappropriate approaches across health and social care, especially for diseases such as dementia and cancer, where comorbidity is the norm rather than the exception (Roda *et al.*, 2017). With the growing interest in personalised medicine, it becomes even more important not only to *classify* or *diagnose* someone as a patient with a certain disorder; its treatment needs a more precise definition of the underlying biology, since different biological origins of the same disease may require (*very*) different treatments (Schnack, 2017).

It really does not matter at all that there exists more than one cogent model for frailty or, in terms of the अनेकान्तवाद parable above, more than one way of 'viewing the elephant'. These models are not actually 'in competition'. The frailty index (FI) is broadly comparable with the frailty phenotype (FP) in predicting risks of future falls, fractures and death. The FP approach is simple to apply in clinical settings, while the FI may be more appropriate as a research tool (Li *et al.*, 2015). The FI and FP agree with each other at a good level of consensus, and both of them predict and discriminate risks of adverse health outcomes significantly in the elderly, which may indicate the flexibility in the choice of frailty model in population-based settings. A general frailty indicator could guide general practitioners (GPs) in directing their care efforts to the patients at highest risk. Lansbury and colleagues (2017) have found it is feasible and acceptable to use the electronic frailty index (eFI). Practice staff ran the eFI reports in five minutes, which they reported was feasible and acceptable. A higher mean eFI in the CGA patients demonstrated construct validity for frailty identification. Practice staff recognised the potential for the eFI to identify the top 2 per cent of vulnerable patients for avoiding unplanned admissions.

Drubbel and colleagues (2013) found that a frailty index based on International Classification of Primary Care-encoded routine healthcare data does predict the risk of adverse health outcomes in an elderly population. Knowledge of the prevalence of frailty can help commissioners and service providers consider how services are delivered within a locality, including hospital care (NIHR Dissemination Centre, 2017). The pressures on the urgent care system have made it difficult to develop proactive approaches to care. It has also led to delays in reactive care, causing patients, especially older people with frailty, to have a poor experience of care, worse clinical and social outcomes, and more rapid deterioration than would be otherwise expected. The three main elements of delivering more proactive care in this report are risk stratification, conducting Comprehensive Geriatric Assessments and creating care plans for multiple eventualities. (The BGS/RCGP report 2016, *Integrated care for older people with frailty: innovative approaches in practice*[3] explains this well.)

The 'sociology of frailty'

Widening the narrative and critique of frailty to beyond the biology of single individuals is essential now, and of vital importance to realising the precise impact of 'intrinsic capacity'. Social relationships – both quantity and quality – affect mental health, health behaviour, physical health and mortality risk. Sociologists have played a central role in establishing the link between social relationships and health outcomes, identifying explanations for this link and discovering social variation (e.g. by gender and race) at the population level. Studies show that social relationships have short- and long-term effects on health, for better and for worse, and that these effects emerge in childhood and cascade throughout life to foster cumulative advantage or disadvantage in health (Umberson and Montez, 2010). The time has come to abandon disease as the focus of medical care. Arguably, the changed spectrum of health, the complex interplay of biological and non-biological factors, the ageing population and the inter-individual variability in health priorities present traditional medical care that is centred on the diagnosis and treatment of individual diseases as, at best, out of date and, at worst, harmful. A primary focus on disease may inadvertently lead to undertreatment, overtreatment or mistreatment (Tinetti and Fried, 2004).

The biomedical model has been critiqued for neglecting the social components, thereby affecting choices in policy and research, and having negative effects on the experience of living with dementia. Other approaches, such as the social model of disability, might be much more relevant to articulating post-diagnostic care and support frameworks for frailty. Chaufan *et al.* (2012), for instance, showed how Alzheimer's disease as we currently know it has actively been constructed as a medicalised condition with a biomedical model of dealing with it. This 'excludes alternative problem definitions', and has led to a 'triumph of cure over care' in policy domains. In the same vein, Moser (2008) studied how Alzheimer's disease has been made to matter in different locations, among which parliamentary politics. She argued that 'pharmaceutical and biomedical versions of the disease [are made] present, visible, strong and dominant', and alternatives are 'made absent, invisible and less real' (pp. 107).

Cognition and frailty

The increased focus on cognitive frailty has been very interesting, not least because this focus at least urges the need for 'frailogists' at least to be holistic. Frailty has been operationalised as a disorder of physical function, but several groups have proposed including cognitive impairment as a frailty criterion. One meeting point of frailty and cognitive decline appears to be delirium. Delirium is an acute disorder of cognitive function, and may be a cognitive manifestation of frailty, where the brain is unable to compensate in the setting of acute systemic stressors. However, delirium is often associated with a decline in physical as well as cognitive functioning. The current frailty criteria, focused on physical function, are necessary for definitional purposes and have made a strong case for using predominantly physical elements. However, it is argued that the functional approach to the geriatric patient makes it difficult to isolate physical from cognitive performance (Quinlan *et al.*, 2011). The contribution of cognitive function to frailty is not well understood, but could be important and warrants further investigation.

The development of 'minimal cognitive impairment' was stimulated first by the clinical awareness of the existence of a grey zone of cognitive impairment that was not captured by any clinical definition and by the rising awareness of dementia as an important area of public health (Petersen *et al.*, 2014). Further, it was reinforced by the emerging clinical need for something beyond the binary diagnosis of the presence or absence of dementia, which could allow an earlier diagnosis and secondary prevention if new treatments were proved efficacious at these early stages. Timely intervention is the optimal strategy for Alzheimer's disease (AD), not only because the patient's level of function will be preserved for a longer period, but also because community-dwelling patients with AD incur less societal cost than those who require long-term institutional placement (Leifer, 2003). This may also be true for some forms of frailty.

The possibility of a prompt, timely diagnosis can refer to different situations: an early diagnosis of dementia (as a cluster of symptoms and signs), a diagnosis of the pathology of Alzheimer's disease in a pre-dementia stage, as well as the diagnosis of Alzheimer's disease before any signs are present at all (called the 'asymptomatic stage') (de Vugt and Verhey, 2013). The discussion of 'activities of daily living' is important. For example, in a recent study (Franse *et al.*, 2017), persons with only primary or secondary education had higher overall frailty and frailty component scores compared to persons with tertiary education. Lower education levels were most consistently associated with higher overall frailty, more morbidities and worse self-rated health. The strongest association was found between primary education and low psychosocial health for persons aged 55–69 years and more instrumental activities of daily living limitations for persons aged 80+ years. Finally, associations between neighbourhood socioeconomic status and frailty (components) also showed inequalities, although less strong. The number of morbidities moderately to strongly mediated the association between socioeconomic indicators and other frailty components.

Communication of risk

The identification of someone's risk of becoming further frail leads onto the equally important question about that communication of risk. There are moral questions about a computer algorithm deducing that someone is 'severely frail', without the patient ever being told, akin to someone with 'incipient dementia' written about him on a neuroimaging investigation without his knowledge. The academic literature about risk now covers a broad spectrum from mathematical analyses to sociological discourses. Both ends of the spectrum deal with uncertainty, but the *quantitative* extreme uses the formal language of probability theory as a tool for analysis, while the *qualitative* end tends to emphasise the political, social and personal responses to perceived hazards (Beck, 2009). Unless the field is careful, practitioners might be unduly precise in their quantitative assessment of frailty, when far more uncertainty exists about how frail somebody is over time. Additional challenges to a fully quantified approach to the analysis of risks can arise from scientific uncertainty, where there are doubts about how the world works or its current state, which in turn produces increased uncertainty about what may happen in the future and what actions might be appropriate now (Spiegelhalter and Riesch, 2011). For instance, does a person who is labelled as 'severely frail' receive then a clear explanation about factors in his or her immediate environment over which he or she can have agency over to reduce his vulnerability?

In communicating chronic risks, there is increasing use of a metaphor that can be termed 'effective-age': the age of a 'healthy' person who has the same risk profile as the individual in question. Popular measures include 'real-age', 'heart-age', 'lung-age' and so on. There are conditions under which the years lost or gained that are associated with exposure to risk factors depends neither on current chronological age, nor the period over which the risk is defined. This is of particular interest to frailty where discussions of 'biological age' rather than 'chronological age' are highly relevant (e.g. Kohanski *et al.*, 2016). These conditions generally hold for all-cause adult mortality, which enables a simple and vivid translation from hazard-ratios to years lost from or gained on chronological age (Spiegelhalter, 2016). Reasonable assumptions, the risks associated with specific behaviours, can be expressed in terms of years gained or lost off your effective age. The idea of effective age appears to be a useful and attractive metaphor to vividly communicate risks to individuals.

Final conclusion

Frailty is most certainly an exciting and challenging field.

This book was proposed to be one of the first substantial single-author syntheses (as a book) of the field of frailty, comprehensively based on a review of the published peer-reviewed literature mainly from the last decade. The bad news is that frailty is inherently shrouded in elements which are as yet rather vague. For example, it is still somewhat unclear if there is a fundamental common biological substrate to various frailty syndromes which causes a person not to recover fully in response to stressors. There are also myths surrounding frailty, such that the phrase 'living well with frailty' sounds inherently contradictory given public perceptions of frailty.

There appears to be little impetus in finding out what 'matters' to people with frailty, such that they are not fully involved in co-design, research or service improvement. There is uncertainty about the extent to which a frailty index might be amenable to change from interventions, but this runs in parallel with a relative under-exploration of measures of resilience and how these affect wellbeing or quality of life. Notwithstanding that, the good news is that frailty is of potential use in working out who might be at most risk for acute admissions to hospital care, or predicting who might do most badly living with concurrent medical comorbidity or undergoing surgical procedures. It would, however, be unfortunate if frailty became entirely defined by what it could be used as a proxy measure for more 'resource intensive' patients and service users, rather than a genuine exploration of how strengths and vulnerabilities could be optimised in a wider ecosystem to benefit people who are frail and care partners.

Certainly, the discussion is now moving towards a critical evaluation of a relationship between assets, deficits and resilience. For example, a 'health assets index' (HAI) has been developed to measure health assets in the hospital setting, based on a systematic review and secondary analysis of the interRAI-Acute Care dataset. Ethical approval has very recently been obtained for a study to determine whether the HAI has predictive validity for mortality and functional decline for hospitalised, frail older adults, given a primary hypothesis that a higher score on the HAI will mitigate the effects of frailty for hospitalised older adults (Gregorevic et al., 2018). But the relationship between assets and deficits needs to be explored. For example, in a recent study of community-dwelling older Thai adults, the "Thai Frailty Index" demonstrated a high prevalence of frailty and predicted mortality but, intriguingly, frail older Thai adults did not earn the protective effect of reducing mortality with higher socioeconomic status (Srinonprasert et al., 2018). An added problem then arises why, if deficits predict mortality so robustly, it might be the case that resilience has little effect. A possible explanation, however, might be provided by acknowledging different time courses of frailty and resilience, thus making resilience not really the 'opposite' of frailty. It is worth noting, therefore, that

Whitson and colleagues (2018) conceptualise resilience as a continuous spectrum that applies across the lifespan; in theory, any person's level of resilience could be quantified at every point in his or her lifetime. In contrast, however, frailty could be thought to happen more near the end of life and represents an extreme part of events within the life course.

Framing the narrative in terms of a 'grey tsunami' might inadvertently channel good intentions of helping certain older people with specific needs into a profoundly 'weaponised policy tool' bringing out ageism at its worst. That is why addressing all stigma, and the root causes of it, is important. It would be helpful if the heterogeneous nature of frailty could be further addressed so that we could identify with much greater clarity the types of patients who might, for example, benefit from a pharmacological approach (e.g. sarcopenia) or who might benefit from a palliative care approach. But, even noting the relative infancy of the field, there seems substantial intrinsic capacity for the future.

Notes

1 https://en.wikipedia.org/wiki/Anekantavada.
2 https://en.wikipedia.org/wiki/Anekantavada.
3 www.bgs.org.uk/pdfs/2016_rcgp_bgs_integration.pdf.

References

Beck U. (2009). *Risk society: towards a new modernity*. London: Sage Publications.

Chaufan CB, Hollister JN, Fox P. (2012). Medical ideology as a double-edged sword: the politics of cure and care in the making of Alzheimer's disease. *Soc. Sci. Med.* 74(5): 788–795.

de Vugt ME, Verhey FRJ. (2013). The impact of early dementia diagnosis and intervention on informal caregivers. *Prog Neurobiol.* 110: 54–62.

Franse CB, van Grieken A, Qin L, Melis RJF, Rietjens JAC, Raat H. (2017). Socioeconomic inequalities in frailty and frailty components among community-dwelling older citizens. *PLoS One.* November 9; 12(11): e0187946. doi:10.1371/journal.pone.0187946. eCollection 2017.

Gregorevic K, Hubbard RE, Peel NM, Lim WK. (2018). Validation of the health assets index in the Australian inpatient setting: a multicentre prospective cohort protocol study. *BMJ Open.* May 10; 8(5): e021135. doi:10.1136/bmjopen-2017-021135.

Kohanski RA, Deeks SG, Gravekamp C, Halter JB, High K, Hurria A, Fuldner R, Green P, Huebner R, Macchiarini F, Sierra F. (2016). Reverse geroscience: how does exposure to early diseases accelerate the age-related decline in health? *Ann N Y Acad Sci.* December; 1386(1): 30–44. doi:10.1111/nyas.13297. Epub 2016 December 1.

Krittanawong C, Zhang H, Wang Z, Aydar M, Kitai T. (2017). Artificial intelligence in precision cardiovascular medicine. *J Am Coll Cardiol.* May 30; 69(21): 2657–64. doi:10.1016/j.jacc.2017.03.571.

Leifer BP. (2003). Early diagnosis of Alzheimer's disease: clinical and economic benefits. *J Am Geriatr Soc.* May; 51(5 Suppl. Dementia): S281–8.

Li G, Thabane L, Ioannidis G, Kennedy C, Papaioannou A, Adachi JD. (2015). Comparison between frailty index of deficit accumulation and phenotypic model to predict risk of falls: data from the global longitudinal study of osteoporosis in women (GLOW) Hamilton cohort. *PLoS One.* March 12; 10(3): e0120144. doi:10.1371/journal.pone.0120144. eCollection 2015.

Moser I. (2008). Making Alzheimer's disease matter: enacting, interfering and doing politics of nature. *Geoforum.* 39(1): 98–110.

NIHR Dissemination Centre. (2017). *Themed review. Comprehensive care: older people living with frailty in hospitals.* www.dc.nihr.ac.uk/themed-reviews/Comprehensive-Care-final. pdf.

Petersen RC, Caracciolo B, Brayne C, Gauthier S, Jelic V, Fratiglioni L. (2014). Mild cognitive impairment: a concept in evolution. *J Intern Med.* March; 275(3): 214–28. doi:10.1111/joim.12190.

Quinlan N, Marcantonio ER, Inouye SK, Gill TM, Kamholz B, Rudolph JL. (2011). Vulnerability: the crossroads of frailty and delirium. *J Am Geriatr Soc.* November; 59(Suppl. 2): S262–8. doi:10.1111/j.1532-5415.2011.03674.x.

Roda A, Michelini E, Caliceti C, Guardigli M, Mirasoli M, Simoni P. (2017). Advanced bioanalytics for precision medicine. *Anal Bioanal Chem.* October 12. doi:10.1007/s00216-017-0660-8. [Epub ahead of print].

Schnack HG. (2017). Improving individual predictions: machine learning approaches for detecting and attacking heterogeneity in schizophrenia (and other psychiatric diseases). *Schizophr Res.* October 24. pii: S0920–9964(17)30649–7. doi:10.1016/j.schres. 2017.10.023. [Epub ahead of print].

Spiegelhalter D. (2016). How old are you, really? Communicating chronic risk through 'effective age' of your body and organs. *BMC Med Inform Decis Mak.* August 5; 16: 104. doi:10.1186/s12911 016-0342-z.

Spiegelhalter D, Riesch H. (2011). Don't know, can't know: embracing deeper uncertainties when analysing risks. *Philos Trans A Math Phys Eng Sci.* December 13; 369(1956): 4730–50. doi:10.1098/rsta.2011.0163.

Srinonprasert V, Chalermsri C, Aekplakorn W. (2018). Frailty index to predict all-cause mortality in Thai community-dwelling older population: a result from a National Health Examination Survey cohort. *Arch Gerontol Geriatr.* May 4; 77: 124–8. doi:10.1016/j. archger.2018.05.002. [Epub ahead of print].

Tinetti ME, Fried T. (2004). The end of the disease era. *Am J Med.* February 1; 116(3): 179–85.

Umberson D, Montez JK. (2010). Social relationships and health: a flashpoint for health policy. *J Health Soc Behav.* 51(Suppl.): S54–66. doi:10.1177/0022146510383501.

Whitson HE, Cohen HJ, Schmader KE, Morey MC, Kuchel G, Colon-Emeric CS. (2018). Physical resilience: not simply the opposite of frailty. *J Am Geriatr Soc.* March 25. doi:10.1111/jgs.15233. [Epub ahead of print].

INDEX

Page numbers in **bold** denote tables, those in *italics* denote figures.